Sewell's Dog's Medical Dictio

Friends of Animals Dogs Names Mullin

- AMBER
- LACEY
- ZUKY
- JO JO
- TERRY
- POINTERS 1 + 2
- ZORRO
- MISSEY
- WHITE TERRIER
- CINDERS
- MAYA
- STICH ⎤
- ELISA ⎥
- HOGAN ⎦
- LURCHER x 2
- LAYA
- LUCY
- MISS BONES.
- SWEEP
- Small TAN/BLACK TERRIER
- BENJI
- DJ + TG
- FRECKLES
- PHOEBEE
- PEPSI
- SILVER
- SOFTIE + her 6 Pups
- TAN SETTER
- COLLIE
- NUGGET
- PEBBLES
- PO - BA

- JACK RUSSELL
- TINY + 4 Pups
- BEAVIS & BUTTHEAD
- PEPPER
- SUSIE
- SPIDER

42 + 10 PUPS

Robert C. White, MRCVS

Sewell's Dog's Medical Dictionary

Routledge & Kegan Paul
London and Henley

First published in 1906 as
The Dog's Medical Dictionary
by Alfred J. Sewell, MRCVS
Third edition, 1932, *revised*
by F. W. Cousens, MRCVS
Fourth edition, 1951, *revised*
by Major Hamilton Kirk, MRCVS
Reprinted with corrections 1962
Fifth edition, *written by*
Robert C. White, MRCVS *published 1976*
by Routledge & Kegan Paul Ltd,
39 Store Street,
London WC1E 7DD *and*
Broadway House,
Newtown Road,
Henley-on-Thames,
Oxon RG9 1EN
and printed in Great Britain by
Western Printing Services Ltd
Bristol
© *Robert C. White, 1976*
No part of this book may be reproduced in
any form without permission from the
publisher, except for the quotation of brief
passages in criticism

ISBN 0 7100 8365 3 (c)
ISBN 0 7100 8366 1 (p)

Contents

	Preface and Acknowledgments	vii
	Introduction	ix
One	**Alphabetical Guide to the Medical Conditions of the Dog**	1
Two	**The Dog in Health**	127
	Canine behaviour patterns	127
	The requirements of the dog in the home or kennel	130
	Canine nutrition	130
	Feeding a dog	133
Three	**Special Diets**	137
	The old dog	137
	The dog with a weakened digestion	137
	The dog with kidney trouble	138
	The diabetic dog	138
	The dog with a bad heart or poor circulation	139
Four	**The Dog when Unwell**	141
	Temperature	141
	Giving tablets	142
	Giving medicine	142
Five	**The First Aid Box**	143
Six	**Weights and Measures**	145

Preface and Acknowledgments

The Dog's Medical Dictionary has been in existence for almost seventy years. During this period it has deservedly become a household necessity for all who have dogs.

Constant revision by a number of authors, each of whom was a specialist in canine care, has maintained the standard of this work. The intention has always been, and is today, to provide a guide to first aid for dogs when qualified help is not immediately available. In addition, in this edition, an indication of the needs of the dog in health is also included. The healthier the dog, the less the need for first aid.

I am grateful to the Hutchinson Publishing Group Ltd for permission to reproduce two Figures from Robert C. White, *The Care of the Family Puppy*.

Introduction

Sewell's Dog's Medical Dictionary is a guide to canine care in health and sickness and, as with all books that cover a wide field, the intelligent reader will use this book with common sense.

Section 1—the alphabetical guide—is intended to be used for reference whenever required. Each entry should be read throughout before acting on the advice contained. Particular attention must be given to the entry with the heading 'Poisoning'.

Sections 2 to 4 are a guide to canine care.

Section 5 outlines the possible contents of a first aid box. These are the minimum that should be available and possibly most of the items listed are normally kept within a home, but it is essential that they are readily to hand in case of an emergency.

Throughout the book, various home treatments and first aid instructions are given. Wherever possible, the dressings or drugs suggested are those mentioned in the list of contents for a first aid box. 'Wound dressing powder' refers to any powder sold for dressing wounds. Acriflavine emulsion is suggested as it is safe, good, and not expensive, but it does have the disadvantage that its yellow colour can stain any material that the dog may brush against. If this is likely to create problems, an alternative such as baby oil can be used.

Canine medicine and surgery are now highly advanced. Modern techniques and drugs are available but should be used only with the guidance of a veterinary surgeon. For this reason, the home treatments mentioned in this book exclude the use of drugs etc. that could do harm if incorrectly used. Thus antibiotics are used to combat infection but, if incorrectly given, can kill, maim, or produce very marked undesirable side-effects.

The principle of home treatment must be that whatever is done must help the dog and not possibly make the condition worse.

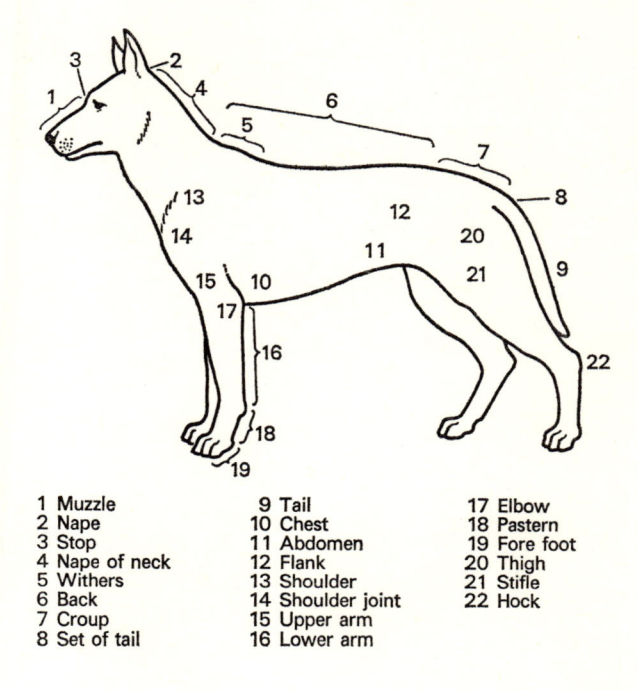

1 Muzzle	9 Tail	17 Elbow
2 Nape	10 Chest	18 Pastern
3 Stop	11 Abdomen	19 Fore foot
4 Nape of neck	12 Flank	20 Thigh
5 Withers	13 Shoulder	21 Stifle
6 Back	14 Shoulder joint	22 Hock
7 Croup	15 Upper arm	
8 Set of tail	16 Lower arm	

Figure 1   Points of the dog

One

Alphabetical Guide to the Medical Conditions of the Dog

Abdominal Pain Pain in the abdomen may be shown by a dog tensing its abdominal muscles, by the adoption of a 'praying attitude' whereby the chest is placed on the ground and the hind quarters are raised, or by the animal objecting to the abdomen being touched.

Just as there are many organs within the abdominal cavity, so there are many causes for the condition. The treatment is dependent on the cause, so the correct diagnosis is of utmost importance and a qualified veterinary surgeon should be consulted as soon as possible. Manual palpation, laboratory tests and X-rays may be required before a definite knowledge of the cause is discovered.

Home treatment should consist of warmth for the dog, rest, and the withholding of water and food. Exercise should be restricted. A small amount (1 teaspoonful) of baby's gripe water can be given every 2 hours.

See also Constipation; Diarrhoea; Rectum, Prolapse of; Vomiting.

Abortion Miscarriage or premature labour does not often occur in the bitch, although it may arise as a result of gross fatigue, injury or severe illness.

Habitual abortion is more likely to occur from an endocrine dysfunction, in which case treatment by injection may be successful. This, however, is not a matter for home treatment, but should be carried out under the advice of a veterinary surgeon.

Certain chronic infections can also cause repeated abortion. Again, qualified assistance is required.

As a general principle, it is inadvisable to try to continue breeding from a bitch that has repeatedly aborted.

The mating of a bitch when the owner does not wish puppies to be born is termed 'misalliance' (q.v.).

Abrasions Sore areas of skin resulting from injury are treated

I

Abscess

by preliminary cleansing, drying with cotton wool and applying zinc or calamine ointment, or by dusting with dry antiseptic powder. Bandaging may be needed to prevent licking (q.v.), but abrasions and wounds heal more readily when not covered. The dog may be muzzled (q.v.) if necessary.

Abscess A collection of pus may occur in any part of the body as a result of infection by a pus-producing organism. The characteristic symptoms are pain, heat and swelling of the affected area. In some cases, the animal's temperature may rise.

An abscess should be 'brought to a head' by hot fomentations or poultices. When this stage is reached, the centre of the abscess should feel soft, and often bursts. If this does not occur, the abscess may be lanced and the contents evacuated. The condition is painful and gentleness is demanded. The opening must not be allowed to heal too quickly and, if the edges cannot be separated easily, it may be necessary to reopen the site. Hot fomentations should be regularly applied for several days to ensure that the wound is clean. Healing should occur from the inside of the abscess.

Where one abscess is present, antibiotic treatment is not often necessary. But where a number of abscesses occur, veterinary advice and treatment are essential.

Care must be taken before treatment is started to ensure that the abscess is not, in fact, a prolapse, hernia or haematoma (qq.v.).

Acariasis, *see* Ear, Inflammation of; Harvest Mites; Mange.

Accidents, *see* Dislocations; Drowning; Fractures; Shock; Wounds, External.

Achondroplasia (Foetal Rickets) An unusual bone formation because the cartilage does not change into bone in the normal way. The long bones are affected before the puppy's birth, so that there is a shortening of the bone.

The condition, which may be hereditary, is normal in heavy, short-legged breeds such as Bassets and Dachshunds. *See* Swimmers.

The treatment is to use corrective external splints, but this is rarely successful. Veterinary advice is needed.

Acidity of Stomach, *see* Dyspepsia; Gastritis.

Acid Milk Can cause digestive upsets in puppies. They tend to lie apart from one another, are cool to the touch, and have distended stomachs. They utter a distinctive plaintive cry.

These indications signify that the bitch is not fit. Her milk

Age, How to Determine

should be tested with blue litmus paper—if it turns red it is a sign that the condition exists and a veterinary surgeon should be consulted.

It is essential that the puppies should be kept warm. They should be given 2 or 3 drops of gripe-water and then fed for a while as orphaned puppies.

See also Hand-Rearing of Puppies.

Acne A localised inflammation of the glands and follicles of the skin, resulting in the formation of pustules which on rupturing discharge a thick sticky pus. This dries into crusty scabs which need soaking and softening with warm antiseptic solutions before removal. They may occur anywhere on the body, but are most commonly seen on the nose, legs and abdomen. They can occur at any age.

Usually causing little pain, they may produce intense irritation which makes the dog scratch excessively. This self-mutilation should be controlled.

As with most skin conditions, veterinary attention is necessary. If this is unobtainable, treatment should consist of baths to keep the skin clean, exercise to reduce boredom (and therefore scratching) and the avoidance of heat. Calamine or zinc lotion should be applied but only in small quantities; if too much is put on, there is the danger of the dog licking the lotion and thus making itself sick.

See also Licking.

Afterbirth Retention, *see* Whelping.

Age (Lifespan) There is no true guide to the possible length of life for a dog, but in most cases it is between 8 and 15 years. As a general principle, the larger the dog, the shorter the expectancy of life, although there are exceptions to this general rule. Especially small dogs are relatively short lived.

Age, How to Determine There is no fixed method for determining the age of a dog. The teeth are the best guide; even they, however, are not a precise indicator. It is generally accepted that the following eruption (or cutting) times are fairly accurate:

Temporary teeth
1st incisors	4–5 weeks
2nd and 3rd incisors	5–6 weeks
canines	3–4 weeks
premolars	4–6 weeks

Aged Dog, Care of

Permanent teeth
- incisors — 4–5 months
- canines — 5 months
- premolars — 4–6 months

Later than this, any estimate of the age of a dog is likely to be very inaccurate.

Aged Dog, Care of The care of the old is really an application of common sense: old dogs are like old people. They are unable to undertake the active life of a younger person or dog. They require less exercise, more warmth and more frequent feeding. Although their sight, hearing and, in fact, all their senses may be restricted, they still require as much affection as they did when young. As a general principle, the aged dog requires a routine that is unaltered and a diet that is plentiful but divided into several meals a day.

See also Section 3.

Albuminuria A condition in which albumin is present in the urine. *See* Kidney Disease.

Allergy The unexpected and unusual reaction to a drug or other substance. This reaction is often manifested as raised areas of the skin where the hairs suddenly begin to stand out. These raised 'plaques' may subside within hours only to be replaced by others in different places. This is most commonly seen in short-haired dogs and is often related to white or light-coloured areas of the skin. Boxers and Short-Haired Dachshunds are most commonly affected.

Treatment consists of keeping the dog cool to reduce the irritation, and therefore the scratching. Antihistamines given by injection or by tablet are used by qualified veterinary surgeons.

In most cases one attack is followed by no sign of recurrence, but where attacks are repeated, it is essential to find the substance that causes this reaction. In humans, it is usual to test for the causative agent, but in dogs, these tests are so expensive that it is more common to record the time of the attacks and, with this as a guide, to attempt to find what food, place or substance seems to induce the attack. Once identified, this should be avoided.

Alopecia True alopecia (or baldness) arising from internal causes must be distinguished from mere asymmetrical loss of hair due to some external agency, as the treatment must always depend on the cause.

Anaesthetics

A common cause is the inability of the body to control the balance of the hormones, the vitamin supply or the nervous system.

As a general principle, the dog should be thoroughly bathed in an anti-parasitic bath, thoroughly dried and the area massaged to stimulate hair growth. A small amount of unsaturated fatty acid (vegetable fat, such as olive oil or margarine) should be added to the diet each week. However, home treatment is not always satisfactory, and veterinary attention must be sought.

So-called 'hair-growing lotions' are of little use. If the cause of the condition can be found, the treatment is more likely to be successful.

Amaurosis, *see* Blindness.

Anaemia A condition of the blood where its ability to carry oxygen is reduced. It can be caused by blood loss or by a reduction in the number of blood cells that are able to carry oxygen. Blood loss can be the result of haemorrhage or of blood-sucking parasites (qq.v.). The reduction of the number of oxygen-carrying cells (red blood cells) may be due to disease, parasites or nutritional deficiencies.

Anaemia due to blood loss is normally quickly corrected by the body as long as the haemorrhage is controlled. The addition of iron and vitamin B to the diet assists this process.

Where anaemia is due to infection, this must be treated before the condition can be corrected. But, again, vitamin B and iron assist recovery.

Parasitic conditions should be treated, and the resultant anaemia will automatically correct itself.

Nutritional deficiencies resulting in anaemia are usually related to lack of iron, cobalt and vitamin B_{12}, although many other deficiencies can indirectly produce the condition.

Virtually all cases will benefit by the administration of iron and arsenic tonic preparations. Raw liver to eat, and liver extracts—either as tablets or in injection form—are of value. The diet should be nourishing, easily digested and may include such items as milk, Virol, Marmite, cod-liver oil, malt extract, etc. Yeast tablets are of value. Sunlight and fresh air combined with the best hygienic conditions assist recovery.

Anaesthetics These can be divided roughly into two groups: local and general.

LOCAL ANAESTHETICS can be applied by injection, by the application

Anal Adenoma

of an ointment, or by a spray. They are used to remove localised pain, to allow painless localised surgery and to block nerves. The latter allows an area of the body to be relieved of all sensation of pain. Local anaesthetics allow the dog to remain conscious and to have control of the body except for the area so treated.

GENERAL ANAESTHETICS are now reasonably safe and reliable. It is sensible to withhold water and food for at least 12 hours before the anaesthetic is given. The risks related to anaesthesia are now greatly reduced, but it must always be remembered that this is a potentially dangerous procedure. The risk is increased in the sick, debilitated, infirm or aged dog.

The use of anaesthetics in any form should at all times be restricted to the veterinary surgeon.

Anal Adenoma This condition is generally seen in male dogs of middle and old age, and consists of tumours that form by the anus. In advanced cases these may bleed and become infected.

Fortunately, this condition usually responds to treatment, given either by injection or by tablet. However, once treatment ceases, there is a tendency for the condition to recur.

Surgical removal of the growth is often successful.

As always, the earlier the treatment is commenced, the greater is the chance of permanent cure.

Anal Glands These are positioned on each side of the anus, under the skin. They contain a thick coloured liquid which can be emptied into the final part of the rectum on sudden movement or when passing a hard motion, and often has a distinctive 'fishy' unpleasant smell.

ABSCESS OF An abscess in the anal gland due to infection should be treated as an abscess. In cases where the condition recurs constantly, it is sensible to consider the surgical removal of the glands.

CONGESTION AND IRRITATION OF

Symptoms Dragging the tail end along the ground (often believed to be due to internal parasites), frequent licking of the anus, suddenly looking at the tail base and putting the tail between the legs as though stung.

Treatment In the simple case, all that is required is to squeeze the glands by pressing upwards and forwards. This evacuates the contents. In some dogs, these glands require attention every three or four weeks.

Analgesia This means the loss of the ability to feel pain without the loss of consciousness or the power of movement, although the latter may be reduced. Analgesia can be induced by freezing, by the local application of liquids or ointment, or by injection. This localised anaesthesia is used for minor surgery; e.g. for the suturing of cuts to the skin.

The injection of a local anaesthetic can also be used to block a nerve and inhibit pain. This should only be undertaken by a veterinary surgeon.
See also Anodyne.

Anaphrodisia A loss of sexual desire in the male, or frigidity in the female. It may arise from dysfunction of one or more hormones, from an unfortunate experience in the past which makes the animal fear the sexual act, from some physical defect or from the results of illness or infection. Treatment depends on the cause and should be carried out by a veterinary surgeon.

However, a different approach to the problem is needed for a virile dog which has been over-used for stud work. Here, rest from mating is indicated, together with good food and exercise. Anything, in fact, that improves the general health will help to increase sexual vigour.

Anodyne A substance or curative measure that soothes pain.

Antibiotics Chemical substances obtained from or produced by living organisms. They have the property when used in certain concentrations of inhibiting the life processes of certain microorganisms.

To be used in medicine, an antibiotic must: 1. be active in the body against one or more types of bacteria, 2. have reliable activity, 3. have low toxicity to tissue, 4. be stable, 5. be not too rapidly excreted. In addition it is desirable that an antibiotic should be active in the presence of body fluids and tissue enzymes and should not give rise to resistant strains of organisms.

The following points are important in the home use of antibiotics. 1. They should be used only when infection is present. 2. The type of antibiotic selected should act against the precise infection present. 3. The dose should be accurately determined. 4. The dose should be given regularly. 5. Treatment should be continued for the full course, even if the infection is overcome at an early stage. Antibiotics should be used only on veterinary advice.

It is possible for a dog to react in an unexpected way to the use

Antibody

of antibiotics (*see* Allergy). When this happens, treatment should be changed.

Examples of antibiotics are penicillin, oxytetracycline, streptomycin and chloramphenicol.

Antibody   A substance found within the body, and formed by the body, which has a specific inhibiting action on an infective organism, toxin or other agent.
See also Immunity; Vaccines.

Antidotes, *see* Poisoning.

Antiseptics   Cleansing agents that stop the growth of bacteria without necessarily killing them. Usually sold in concentrated form and therefore requiring dilution before use. If used in too strong a concentration, they can damage tissue. Many antiseptics can be used as disinfectants if the strength is increased. (A disinfectant is a preparation that can kill infective organisms.)

Hydrogen peroxide and the various hyperchlorite solutions (such as Eusol, Deosan, Milton, etc.) are examples of unstable antiseptics—those that must be used only when freshly prepared.

Another excellent, safe and non-irritant antiseptic is acriflavine, its disadvantage being its property of staining everything yellow. A 1 per cent solution of Crystal Violet or Gentian Violet is also effective but, again, has staining properties.

Common salt (a 5 ml spoonful to 0·5 litre of boiled water) is useful as a wound lotion.

Dettol is non-irritating and non-toxic and retains its activity in the presence of pus, etc.

The use of mercurial or coal-tar preparations and of iodoform should be avoided; if they are absorbed or licked, poisoning may result. Whatever antiseptic is used, it is essential to read and follow the instructions supplied on, or with, the container.

Antiserum, *see* Immunity.

ANUS (*see also* Anal)

External Occlusion of   A common condition seen in long-haired breeds. The anal opening is completely blocked by a mass of dried faeces attached to the hairs around the anus. Great discomfort and pain are produced, while the smell of the mass is unmistakable.

The removal of such a mass requires the greatest patience and deftness of manipulation, as generally little more than 1 or 2 mm separate it from the skin, to which it is held by fine hairs. All these

Anus

must be cut with scissors, care being taken not to cut the skin. The discomfort of the condition usually makes the dog restless. It is often best to soak the mass with warm water before attempting its removal. Neat 10 vols hydrogen peroxide poured over the mass will in some cases help to separate it from the skin.

Fissure of A small painful crack or ulcer situated just within the anus and seldom involving more than the mucous membrane.
Symptoms Pain during and after passing a motion. There may be blood or pus on the motion.
Treatment Evert the margin of the anus and clean gently. A soothing ointment should be applied.

This condition is often difficult to heal and can be misdiagnosed. Where response is not good (healing within 2 or 3 days), veterinary advice must be obtained.

Fistula A condition where deep abscesses occur round the anus. Seen more commonly in Alsatians. Is often difficult to heal and in many cases requires surgical treatment. Veterinary attention should be sought.

Imperforate A relatively rare condition where a puppy is born without the anal opening. The owner's attention is drawn to the fact by the dog's continuous straining to defecate without effect, and by the swelling which occurs at a point corresponding to the normal anus.

Treatment is surgical and must be performed by a veterinary surgeon.

Irritation of Treatment depends on the cause, which may be parasitism (worms), enlarged prostate glands, anal gland conditions, anal fistula, chronic diarrhoea, or a foreign body lodged in the rectum (qq.v.). As a first aid measure a soothing ointment should be applied to the area. A finger inserted into the rectum will determine if a foreign body is present. The area should be kept clean.

Pruritus Ani (irritation of the skin surrounding the anus) This condition is caused by swollen and inflamed anal glands, enlargement of the prostate gland, anal adenoma or localised inflammation (qq.v.).

The skin around the anus is inflamed and red. The dog tends to rub the buttocks and anus along the ground, and to lick the anal region; it is often irritable. When walking, it may sit down suddenly as though stung; when sitting, it may suddenly jump, and look at the tail region.

Aphrodisia

The anal glands should be emptied by pressure upwards and forwards exerted on each side of the anus. The area should be kept clean, and a soothing cream applied. When healing has started, talcum powder should be used in place of the cream to dry the skin.

Aphrodisia (excess libido) A condition seen mainly in male dogs, which may result from frustrated sexual desire, lack of exercise or some endocrine imbalance. For such animals, the obvious treatment is more work and a stimulating life. The work can be provided by increased exercise (perhaps to the point of fatigue), while the diet should include more fish and biscuit and less red meat. Sedatives (e.g. bromides) can be used for short periods, but should not be administered indefinitely.

Castration (q.v.) is a drastic but effective form of treatment. There is no reason why this should not be considered as, once the immediate effects of the operation are over, the dog is healthy and happy.

Synthetic oestrogens will control excessive sexual drive but their use has disadvantages and these should be fully understood before treatment commences. Naturally this treatment can only be prescribed by a veterinary surgeon.

Apoplexy, *see* Stroke.

APPETITE

Decreased It is essential to distinguish between actual loss of appetite and the inability to eat although hungry. The latter may be due to some painful lesion in the mouth or throat (e.g. an ulcer, toothache, or the result of an infection), or a physical obstruction such as a bone which has become lodged in the throat or on or between the teeth.

Old age, injury and ill-health often produce a decrease in appetite.

Treatment must depend on the cause. If there is any doubt, the advice of a veterinary surgeon should be obtained.

A simple and often beneficial way to promote appetite is to administer yeast. This, together with an interesting and varied diet, will help. Finally, if another (healthy) dog can be fed in front of the patient, the sense of competition will often stimulate appetite.

Depraved The animal eats stones, coal, manure, etc., and the suggested causes include teething, worms, indigestion, rickets, the lack of salt or one or more essential vitamins in the diet, or even actual hunger. Puppies exhibit this symptom rather more than adult dogs, and it is always wise to treat for worms and to ensure that the diet contains some common salt, calcium and a vitamin supplement.

Puppies sometimes chew wood, bones, coke or coal to relieve irritation of the gums. Grass-eating (q.v.) is not a sign of a depraved appetite.

Where a habit has been developed, it is sensible to dust the object of the depraved appetite with cayenne pepper or powdered bitter aloes and then offer it to the dog. The taste may be so unpleasant that the dog will be deterred. Naturally, all possible care should be taken to ensure that the object of this habit is kept out of the dog's way for as long as possible, to enable it to forget the whole thing.

Muzzling the dog (q.v.), when at liberty, will mechanically prevent the habit.

Increased While a ravenous appetite is not necessarily a sign of ill-health, especially in rapidly growing puppies or lactating bitches, one has to draw the line between what is normally expected in the way of food requirements, and what has become an abnormal or insatiable hunger. A common cause is internal parasitism, which should be treated by appropriate methods. Other possible causes include Pseudo-Diabetes (a pancreatic disease) and true Diabetes Mellitus (qq.v.).

Arthritis Inflammation of a joint, or disease involving a joint; more strictly, articular inflammation. It may be due to effects of injury, infection or malfunction of the joint. It can be classed as acute or chronic.

Symptoms The joint may be swollen and painful. The dog attempts to avoid the use of the joint, is often lame, and in cases where a joint of a limb is involved may be unable to put that foot to the ground. It is essential to ensure that no fracture exists; an X-ray is indicated.

Treatment During acute inflammation, rest and warmth are necessary but veterinary treatment is also necessary. Pain-relieving drugs and anti-inflammatory agents are often used. The joint may be supported by a bandage. Where infection exists, this must be treated. Temporary relief may be afforded by giving one-quarter to one 300 mg tablet of soluble aspirin (q.v.) every 4 hours.

Artificial Eyes, Limbs and Teeth

Where treatment is succeeding, it is sensible to continue it for a number of days after recovery appears to be complete. In chronic cases, recovery may not be completely achieved.

If the dog is over-weight, reduce the amount of food given and thus enforce a valuable weight loss.

Artificial Eyes, Limbs and Teeth These prosthetic aids can be made and used for canine patients. However, their use is limited, partly due to their cost, and partly due to the problem of ensuring that the dog adjusts to their use.

Individual teeth are sometimes inserted into the jaw of a dog that has lost a tooth through injury. This is usually successful and has been used for working dogs that require a strong bite.

Artificial Insemination A method of transference of the male semen to the female without sexual intercourse. Occasionally used in dogs but of no practical use to the non-specialist dog-owners.

Artificial Respiration When a drowned dog stops breathing, hold it up by the hind legs with the head hanging down to allow the water to escape from the lungs. Speed is essential. As soon as the water has ceased to run out of the mouth, lay the dog on its side, pull the tongue out as far as possible and commence artificial respiration. This means placing the palms of both hands (except with minature breeds, when only one hand is used) over the chest surface, i.e. the rib area, and rhythmically and slowly press and release, so that the air is driven out of the lungs and then allowed to re-enter on the release of pressure. This cycle should be repeated about thirty times a minute for small dogs and about twenty times a minute for large dogs.

Artificial respiration should not be performed jerkily or roughly, the object being to drive out residual air, and to permit its re-entry, in time and manner as nearly as possible approaching the normal.

This routine must be continued as long as the heart is still beating—the heart action may at first be so feeble that it cannot be detected by feeling the chest. As time goes by it is to be hoped that the strength of the heart beat will increase until it can be felt and that respiration will restart without the need of external help. If you are alone, continue, and stay with the dog for 2 hours before leaving it to seek help.

If the heart seems definitely to have stopped beating, a regular sharp tap on the chest near the heart may stimulate action. If this is going to be effective, the beat will resume within a few seconds.

Asthma

This does not always work, but is well worth trying. If the heart restarts within 30 seconds, then recommence artificial respiration. If no beat occurs within this time, I regret that you should stop your efforts.

Quite apart from manual artificial respiration, the use of certain fumes stimulates respiration. The fumes of ammonia, carbon dioxide or smelling-salts, if placed near the dog's nose for a second, often create normal breathing.

Ice held against the nostrils often proves helpful.

Do not attempt to make the animal swallow if it is unconscious or collapsed.

Ascariasis or **Ascaridiasis** (intestation with roundworms), *see* Parasites, Internal.

Ascites (Abdominal Dropsy), *see* Dropsy.

Asepsis A surgical term to describe a principle employed during the preparation and conduct of an operation when, instead of relying upon the use of germicides to avoid infection, one autoclaves or otherwise destroys infection on all surgical instruments, dressings, gloves, etc. The object is to cleanse and sterilise everything likely to touch the animal so that no germs remain to infect it. Needless to say, the animal's skin is clipped, shaved, scrubbed and disinfected very thoroughly, and all parts of the limb or body not immediately concerned in the operation are draped with sterile towels. Aseptic after-treatment of the operation wound is exceedingly important if the wound is to heal without infection.

Asphyxia (Failure of respiration) This may be caused by a number of conditions such as carbon monoxide poisoning, overdosage with narcotics, drowning, bee-stings causing swelling of the throat, foreign bodies in the throat or oesophagus, haemorrhage (qq.v.).

Wherever possible, the cause should be discovered and removed immediately. Artificial respiration (q.v.) should be applied if needed. The advice of a veterinary surgeon should be sought, but immediate first aid is also essential.

Aspirin A drug in tablet form used to control pain and other aspects of ill-health. In the dog, it can cause vomiting. The soluble form is better accepted. Can be used to relieve muscular pain.

Asthma The name given to respiratory difficulty, often of sudden or spasmodic occurrence. Probably most cases are caused by a chronic bronchitis. Others are due to some kind of peripheral irritation associated with the very sensitive bronchial mucous membranes. Cardiac asthma arises from poor circulation caused by heart malfunction and is often encountered in elderly dogs.

During an attack, the dog should be placed in such a position that it can obtain a plentiful supply of fresh air. When a dog is unconscious, the head should be raised and the tongue pulled as far as possible out of the mouth to ensure that the passage to the lungs is unobstructed. Steam (not hot enough to burn), the fumes of Friar's Balsam or Vick will often help. The advice of a veterinary surgeon should be obtained and the cause determined. Once the attack is over, it is essential to treat the cause to try to prevent a recurrence.

Atavism, *see* Hereditary Abnormalities.

Ataxia A muscular or nervous disorder involving the voluntary movements of progression. The legs may be picked up and carried forward, as in walking, but they are not put down in such positions as will permit the body balance to be maintained. The animal staggers in consequence. There are numerous causes and variable methods of treatment, but this is not a condition that can be treated by the amateur. Every case has to be treated on its merits and professional advice is essential.

Atrophy The degeneration or shrinking of tissues due to interference with their nutrition or nerve supply or to disuse. This is well illustrated by the muscles of a leg that tend to shrink if the limb is enclosed in a plaster cast for some time. Treatment is directed to the stimulation of the blood and/or nerve supply of the part affected. Stimulation may be provided by hand massage, exercise, hot fomentations, heat rays, etc. Drugs to stimulate repair and to strengthen the tissues are used by qualified practitioners.

Aural Diseases, *see* Ear.

Babesiosis, Canine A disease, caused by *Babesia canis* and *B. gibsoni*, caught from the bite of an infected tick. Widespread in warmer parts of the world.

Symptoms High temperature, depression, rapid breathing, loss of appetite, rapid pulse, weakness and staggering. Anaemia develops and jaundice may be present. Diagnosis confirmed by examination of blood sample.

Treatment The dog should be treated to remove any ticks. Warmth, rest and veterinary advice are essential.

Bacillus A micro-organism having a rod-shaped appearance when seen under the microscope. Examples of some of the diseases caused by bacilli are anthrax, tuberculosis and some forms of colitis.

Back-Ache This condition is shown by the stiff movements of the dog, unwillingness to turn round or to climb stairs. Pain is present which causes the unwillingness to move. The dog may cry when the back is touched. Causes may be actual injury, a disc lesion, infection, or a lowering of resistance due to over-exertion, cold or damp. May be associated with kidney disease (including leptospirosis (q.v.)) or muscular rheumatism.

The diagnosis must not be at fault, and will be helped by a urine test if nephritis is suspected, and by X-ray if injury to the spine is considered possible.

Soluble aspirin, codeine, and similar analgesic tablets often prove a useful means of home treatment where actual injury is not present. Rest and warmth are essential.

Bacterium A term applied to any microscopic organism, no matter what its shape. It is synonymous with 'germ', 'micro-organism' and 'microbe'.

Bad Breath, *see* Breath, Foul.

Balanitis, *see* Penis.

Baldness, *see* Alopecia.

Bark, Hoarse (*see also* Laryngitis; Pharyngitis) In countries where rabies (q.v.) is present, it is necessary to ensure that the alteration of the bark is not a sign of that disease.

Barley Water A useful demulcent drink which is prepared by simmering 60 g of pearl barley in 1 litre of water for 2 hours, and straining while still hot. No lemon is added. The drink is offered slightly warmed. Useful in cases of diarrhoea, urinary disease, sore throat and mouth, fever, and when the appetite is reduced.

Barrenness, *see* Sterility.

Baths If a dog is combed and brushed regularly, frequent baths are unnecessary. Combing prevents matting of the hair, while brushing removes dust and surface dirt. Bathing tends to soften hair and, if carried out too often, may weaken it.

However, a twice-yearly bath, or whenever the dog is dirty or has an unpleasant smell, is sensible.

Probably the easiest way is to stand the dog in a depth of 5–10 cm of warm water (about $35°$ C is ideal) in the bath. Using a mug or

Bed-Sores

sponge, pour the water over the dog and apply dog shampoo thoroughly, not forgetting the legs and tail. Then rinse off the lather, using clean warm water. It is essential that all the residual shampoo be removed.

If a medicated bath is indicated, it is essential that the chemical or drug involved is used in the correct dilution. Some of these liquids are to be rinsed off, others are not, so the directions must be carefully read and followed.

Once bathed, a dog must be dried and then kept warm for a time. It is wrong to let a damp dog lie in the cold.

Small dogs can be bathed in the same way in the kitchen sink.

Bed-Sores These sores are caused by pressure when a dog lies on a hard surface for long periods, and are seen most commonly in the larger breeds. They are usually to be seen on the hips, hock, elbow and shoulder, but they can occur on any part of the body, depending on the dog's position when lying.

Treatment If at all possible, the cause should be removed; i.e. if the dog lies on a specific hard surface, this should be padded with several layers of blanket. The sores should be cleaned with warm water, dried gently and dressed—if hard, acriflavine emulsion can be used; if moist, the sore can be sprinkled with a wound dressing powder. Any infection must be treated. Open sores are better left unbandaged to allow the air to reach the site, provided that they can be kept clean and the dog cannot interfere with the damaged tissue.

If the sores are large, infected or not responding to treatment, veterinary advice must be obtained.

Bee Stings, *see* Stings.

Benign Tumours, *see* Tumours.

Biliousness A name sometimes given to temporary gastric upset with slight vomiting. Food and water should be avoided for 24 hours. Recovery should be quick. If not, or if the condition constantly recurs, veterinary advice should be obtained.

Bites A wound caused by the bite of a dog or cat can be either a deep puncture wound or a tear in the skin. The area should be cleaned and the hair clipped to allow examination of the wound. Where the bite is a deep puncture, it is essential to ensure that healing occurs from the bottom of the wound—the puncture in the skin should not otherwise be allowed to heal, as this might predispose to abscess formation. Small tears are often kept clean

Bladder

but not sutured, as the danger of infection is always present. Large tears require suturing.

Bites must be bathed regularly to keep dirt, discharges and hair away. Wound dressing powder is an ideal help towards healing.

Care must be taken to ensure that the animal does not lick the wound or increase the damage. A dressing can be applied if needed. Muzzling the dog (q.v.) at times is occasionally necessary but does not always stop the interference with the wound.

If in doubt, or if the dog shows signs of poor appetite, high temperature, or the wound is not healing, veterinary advice should be obtained. Large wounds must have veterinary attention.

Biting Some dogs are naturally aggressive, not only to other dogs and to cats, but also to human beings. It is now believed that this behaviour pattern is usually the result of bad management of the animal in the early part of life (*see* Canine Behaviour Patterns in Section 2). It is equally true that a good dog can be made into a difficult animal by bad management at any age. It is essential that a dog should be treated with kindness throughout its life. Training will often help to control a dog that shows signs of aggression, as this provides a form of mental exercise. Training, however, is not just a question of making a dog do what it is told; it is really a means to make a dog want to obey. Training should be carried out with other dogs under the supervision of an experienced trainer. Training classes are organised throughout the country. The address of the one nearest to your home can usually be obtained from the RSPCA or from the Kennel Club.

Castration is often effective in reducing the male dog's desire to fight or bite.

It is worth remembering that it is rare for a dog actually to be born bad tempered; rather, it is the management of the dog that produces aggressive tendencies.

Black Stools This is usually a symptom of haemorrhagic gastro-enteritis (q.v.).

Black Tongue, *see* Tongue.

BLADDER

Distended The cause is the obstruction of the outflow of urine or paralysis of the muscular part of the bladder. An obstruction may be due to a stone or a stricture of the passage from the bladder. Veterinary treatment is essential, as the condition can be extremely serious.

Bleeding

Irritability of This condition is shown by the dog continuously straining and attempting to pass water. Some urine is produced, often containing signs of blood. The causes are either inflammation of the bladder or mechanical obstruction of the urethra. Veterinary treatment is essential. As a first aid measure—pending the arrival of qualified help—the owner may give 200–600 mg of hexamine every 4 hours.
See also Cystitis.

Paralysis of In this condition, the dog does not pass water in the normal way, but allows the urine to dribble away slowly, as the bladder walls are incapable of exerting pressure to force the urine out of the body. The bladder remains full—it is only the 'overflow' that escapes.

The bladder can usually be emptied by grasping the abdominal wall and exerting gentle and even pressure on the bladder. The appearance of a steady flow of urine from the penis or vulva will demonstrate that no mechanical obstruction exists.

The bladder should be emptied twice daily, completely and thoroughly and every effort made to ensure that when this is carried out the bladder is completely emptied as any urine remaining can predispose to cystitis.

A catheter can be used, but unskilled persons are strongly advised to avoid this method of bladder emptying as it can produce additional inflammation and even infection.

Bleeding, *see* Haemorrhage.
Blepharitis, *see* Eyelid.
Blindness (loss of sight) There are many causes, including damage to the eye itself, to the retina, to the optic nerve or to the brain. It may be temporary—e.g. after injury where the damage is repairable, or permanent.

Blindness can be a hereditary condition in dogs, where the retina degenerates at a certain age (*see* Hereditary Abnormalities, Progressive Retinal Atrophy).

Amaurosis is the name given to blindness when there is no visible change in the eye when the dog's head is examined casually. The term is not now frequently used.

If a dog begins to go blind, it is not uncommon for the owner not to be aware of this fact for some time as the dog is able to use its senses of smell and hearing to compensate for the gradual loss of sight.

Treatment, if possible, depends on the cause, and the advice of a veterinary surgeon is essential.
See also Blue Eye.
Blisters These are sacs seen under the skin which contain a watery serum with or without blood; they may be caused by blows or burns. Blisters should not be opened but should be dressed with acriflavine emulsion, covered by a gauze pad, and bandaged. Occasionally they occur on a site it is impossible to bandage, in which case they should be dressed, but left without a covering.
Bloat This condition occurs in young puppies. The abdomen is excessively distended and the puppy usually cries with a loud piercing sound. A small amount (2-3 drops) of baby's gripe-water should be given to ease the collection of wind. Expert advice should be sought if recovery is not rapid.
See also Anus, Imperforate.
Blood A red fluid which has the functions of nourishing the tissues of the body, aiding in their growth and repair, and transporting many substances within the body.
See also Haemorrhage.
Blood-Poisoning A popular name for septicaemia (q.v.).
Blood Transfusion The transfer of blood from one animal (the donor) to another (the recipient). Normally used in cases of acute haemorrhage or shock (qq.v.). Care has to be taken to ensure that the recipient is able to accept the donor's blood, as the many blood groups differ slightly from each other and in some cases react adversely when inter-mixed.
Blue Eye, *see* Eye.
Boils, *see* Abscesses.
Bones, Broken, *see* Fractures.
BOWEL
Foreign Bodies in In general, it is a dangerous practice to give dogs rabbit, chicken, or chop bones as these may become lodged within the digestive tract and cause trouble. Puppies may pick up and swallow stones, buttons, nails, needles, etc., and even though these may reach the stomach and intestines safely, they may cause an obstruction there.

Where this has happened, the dog often shows signs of abdominal discomfort, vomiting, restlessness and sometimes blood from the anus. It passes no more motions after a while. It is sometimes possible to feel the mass of the obstruction through the abdominal

Bowel

wall when the hands are placed each side of the dog. Whenever this condition is suspected, an X-ray is indicated. It is dangerous to give any form of purgative, indeed it is probably better to withhold all food, water and medicine until advice is obtained. The faeces, if any, should be examined to find if any unusual content is present—this may assist the veterinary surgeon when he is examining the dog.

Inflammation of (Enteritis)
Causes Improper, or too much, food; organic or mineral poisons (q.v.); sudden severe changes in the weather; certain diseases such as distemper, leptospirosis, coccidiosis, septicaemia, tuberculosis; localised infection; worms; indigestion; foreign bodies; chills (qq.v.) or irritants.

Symptoms Pain in abdomen, restlessness; if a puppy, it whines and cries; generally diarrhoea with some mucus but possibly constipation; often vomiting at frequent intervals. Seldom a rise in temperature unless the condition is very acute or caused by a disease. The pulse rate is often increased.

Enteritis may be accompanied by marked tenderness when the abdomen is touched; the muscles of the abdomen may be tensed and the back arched.

Veterinary advice is essential. As a first aid measure give 5–15 drops of Chlorodyne in a little water every 3 hours. Withhold solid food and limit the water intake.

Invagination of One part of the bowel telescopes into another, thus causing an obstruction. It is a very serious condition, as the malpositioned part has a restricted blood supply. If surgical treatment is carried out as quickly as possible, the chance of recovery is good.

The symptoms are similar to those of foreign bodies swallowed (q.v.) but the swelling can often be felt within the abdominal cavity. It occurs most commonly in young puppies and may be associated with a prolapse of the rectum (q.v.).

Stoppage of The collection of faeces within the bowel, which becomes hard and impossible to pass out of the body.

It is wrong to conclude that a dog has a bowel stoppage just because it has not passed a motion for a given period. A change in the amount of exercise, the diet, or even in the house may cause an alteration in its habits. Foreign bodies and invagination of the bowel (qq.v.) can result in similar symptoms.

A liquid diet, with liquid paraffin, will help. An enema of warm soapy water (good white soap) can often bring quick relief.

BRAIN

Concussion of This is usually the result of a blow on the head due to a car accident or a fall when the function of the brain is disturbed although the skull may not be fractured. Initially the dog is usually unconscious. Later, it starts to move but has lost the full control of its movements.

In many cases the symptoms gradually pass off until full control is regained.

No attempt must be made to give anything by mouth while the dog is unconscious. Where respiration is affected, smelling salts or ammonia fumes can be placed for a few moments by the dog's nose. The dog's body should be well covered and it should be kept in a warm room. Constant supervision is required when the dog attempts to move to ensure that additional injuries do not occur due to lack of co-ordination.

Congestion of An excessive amount of blood in the blood vessels of the brain. It may be the result of acute infection, poisons, changes in the blood vessels of the brain, heat, or parasites.

The symptoms often are excitement, howling, rapid breathing and uncontrolled movements. Each attack lasts for a period, followed by rest, then a recurrence of the symptoms.

The dog should be isolated, kept in a cool darkened room away from noise or any form of stimulus. Ice or cold water can be applied to the head. Veterinary attention is required.

Haemorrhage, *see* Stroke.

Inflammation of This condition may be a sequel to congestion of the brain, or it may arise from injuries to the head, exposure to extreme heat, excessive fatigue, tumours, distemper, tuberculosis, etc.

In the early stages the dog may dislike being watched and hide under furniture. It is restless, whines frequently, but is not aggressive. This stage usually soon passes. It then becomes unresponsive and stupid, staring into space, perhaps pressing its head against a wall or walking in circles (always in one direction only). Later there may be blindness, deafness or paralysis, or a combination of these symptoms.

Quiet, warmth and security are essential. Veterinary help is needed.

Breasts, Inflamed, *see* Mastitis.

BREATH
Foul Breath This is usually associated with deterioration of the teeth (caries, scale, ulcerated gums or mouth surfaces, qq.v.), for which veterinary dental treatment is indicated. Other causes may be gastro-intestinal upsets, kidney trouble or infection. In true diabetes (q.v.), there is a distinctive smell of acetone.

In the Spaniel, one may notice an extremely unpleasant odour which might be thought to be associated with the breath but which in fact arises from an ulceration of the outer surfaces of the lower lip. This occurs in the deep creases seen in this breed which fill with saliva and then become infected. Creases thus affected should be cleaned, washed with a 10 vol. hydrogen peroxide solution, dried and powdered with a wound dressing powder.

In all cases of true foul breath, the cause must be found and treated.

Loss of Breath Often the result of poor heart action, when insufficient blood is passed through the lungs. There may be an associated cough. This condition is more often seen in older dogs, or in those recovering from a prolonged illness. Anaemia (however caused), diseases of the lungs and unusual exercise may also produce this effect.

Breathing Difficulty in Short-Nosed Breeds
Causes Short nose, elongated soft palate, malformation of the nostrils.
Treatment Usually surgical; veterinary advice essential.

Breeding, to Prevent Keep the bitch under strict control when she is in season to ensure that she cannot be mated; or surgical removal of the ovaries and uterus (*see* Spaying). An injection to prevent her coming into season, or tablets for the same purpose, can be obtained after advice from a veterinary surgeon.
See also Misalliance.

Breeding Cycle of the Bitch Under normal conditions the bitch comes into season at 6–12 months of age, and thereafter regularly at intervals of about 6 months. The actual season lasts for approximately 3 weeks but the bitch will accept a dog for mating only for a few days during the second week.

During the season, the vulva swells, and a blood-stained discharge occurs. At the 10th–12th day, this is usually reduced.
See also Oestrus.

Burns and Scalds

Bronchitis The term used for inflammation of the bronchi or windpipes. This condition may be caused by exposure, sudden changes of temperature, misdirection of liquid medicine or food, inhalation of poisonous gases or dust, infection, or poor circulation. Often associated with a dry, short, intermittent cough. Treatment consists of controlling infection, avoiding over-exercise and extremes of temperature, and the housing and nursing of the dog in an area that is warm, dry, well ventilated but without draughts. Inhalants often give relief; a teaspoonful of Friar's Balsam added to a bowl containing 0·5 litre of hot water produces a steam which can be breathed.

It is advisable in all cases to ask a veterinary surgeon to determine the cause and to advise the best treatment.

Brown Mouth, *see* Gum.

Bruises These are areas of the body discoloured by blood filtering into the tissues following an injury. In nearly all cases no treatment is needed. The discoloration gradually changes and disappears within 7-10 days. Licking or rubbing of the affected part should be stopped (*see* Licking).

If the area affected is extremely swollen, expert advice should be obtained in case other injuries are present.

Burns and Scalds A burn is an injury caused by dry heat, e.g. a fire or a piece of hot material. A scald is an injury caused by moist heat, e.g. boiling water, tar or fat. Special forms of burns can be caused by certain chemicals, excessive cold or electric currents.

The severity of the symptoms will depend on the intensity of the heat applied, the length of time the dog remains in contact with it and the area of skin involved. All burns affecting more than 10 per cent of the body surface must be regarded as severe and treated with great care. Shock is a major complicating factor.

Treatment The first step must always be to remove the cause of the burn if it is still present. If this is an electric current, this should be turned off before the animal is touched. Any burning hair should be instantly cooled with water.

In case of shock, or if the burn is extensive, skilled attention must be obtained. The following first aid measures can be carried out. Place the dog in a warm bed with hot-water bottles or an electric blanket. The burn should be gently cleaned. If it is contaminated by straw, grass or other matter, this may be soaked off using warm water and soap. Provided the dog does not lick or bite the wound it should be left uncovered and undressed until expert help arrives. If, however, the dog may do further damage, the area should be covered with a gauze pad or clean white cloth and gently bandaged. This pad or cloth should be soaked in tea, acriflavine emulsion or tannic acid jelly.

BURNS BY ACID These are treated by flooding the area with water and neutralising with dilute ammonia or bicarbonate of soda.

BURNS BY ALKALIS These should be washed with warm water and a weak solution of vinegar or lemon juice.

SCALDS The treatment of scalds is the same as that for burns. It should, however, be noted that a scald may not destroy hair when it damages the skin, so the visible signs may not be so easily observed at first sight. Care must therefore be taken to determine the extent of the scald—it can be detected by the increased colours of the areas affected.

Bursitis Inflammation of a synovial bursa, often at exposed points such as the elbow and hock, caused by injury or by pressure at these points when the animal is lying down. They are commoner in larger dogs. The swellings are of varying size and severity, and often very resistant to treatment. Veterinary attention is required.

Caesarean Section, *see* Whelping.

Calculus (also known as a 'stone') This is a solid mass of crystals of various salts, usually urates, oxalates, carbonates, or phosphates of calcium or magnesium. Stones may form in any part of the urinary system, but are most commonly found in the bladder or gallbladder.

The main symptom is the frequent passing of urine, which is often blood-stained.

In the male, renal stones, if small, may enter the urinary passage or urethra and become lodged in the canal just behind the bone in the penis where the passage is smallest. If the stone is round, it acts like a cork in a bottle, and the dog is unable to pass water. If it has an irregular shape, the dog can pass small amounts of water, often highly coloured, after severe straining.

The bitch is able to pass small stones without undue difficulty.

To determine if a stone is causing such an obstruction in the male, an X-ray or the passage of a catheter (q.v.) is required.

Calculi in the bladder can sometimes be felt if the hands are placed on each side of the abdominal wall and gentle pressure used. X-rays will confirm the diagnosis.

Treatment In most cases surgical removal of the stone or stones is essential. Occasionally drugs can assist.

If a dog has suffered from this condition, the trouble is likely to recur. It is sensible to have the stone analysed in a laboratory to find its composition. Once this is known, a change of diet may help to prevent further attacks. In the same way it is possible to determine what course of medication would be most likely to prevent a recurrence.

Cancer, *see* Tumours.
Canicola Fever, *see* Leptospirosis.
Canine Virus Hepatitis This is a widespread virus disease of dogs. It can occur in various forms, varying from the *hyperacute* where the dog may be found dead without a previous illness, to the *subclinical* where no symptoms occur.

Diagnosis and treatment must be carried out by a veterinary surgeon.

Infection is spread mainly in the urine, and the risk of this continues for a long time after recovery. All exercise yards, pens and kennels which may carry infection must be kept clean. Every part must be thoroughly scrubbed with a hot strong solution of washing soda as often as possible and then left for 24 hours, being finally thoroughly rinsed with fresh water to remove the remaining soda.

Some dogs, during the period of recovery from canine virus hepatitis, develop a dense opacity of the surface of one or both eyes. *See* Blue Eye; *see also* Vaccines.

Canker of the Ear, *see* Ear.
Capped Elbow or Hock, *see* Bursitis.
Car Sickness, *see* Travel Sickness.
Carbuncle, *see* Abscess.
Caries of Bone This term is not now generally employed; at one time it was used to refer to necrosis of bone.
Caries of Teeth, *see* Teeth.
Castration The surgical removal of the essential sex organs. This term is normally used in connection with the male dog, 'spaying' (q.v.) being used for a bitch. The testicles of the male are removed, and the uterus and ovaries of the female.

Cataract

This operation must be carried out by a veterinary surgeon—there is little risk and no aesthetic objection. It can be done at any age and, while the ideal age is debatable, most surgeons prefer the dog to be 4 to 5 months old.

Cataract, *see* Eye.

Catarrh The inflammation of a mucous membrane such as the lining of the nose, cheeks, bronchi, stomach, etc. associated with the secretion of mucus. The condition is named according to the organ or part implicated, e.g. nasal catarrh, gastric catarrh. It arises from exposure to cold or damp, careless washing, irritant dust, or, more usually, from infection.

Catheter An instrument which can be passed through the penis or vagina into the bladder and used to remove urine which the animal cannot voluntarily pass. Catheterisation is a procedure which requires knowledge, skill, and a particular attention to surgical cleanliness, and should never be attempted by the amateur.

Cerebellar Ataxia, *see* Ataxia.

Cerebral Congestion, *see* Brain, Congestion of.

Cerebral Haemorrhage, *see* Stroke.

Chemotherapy The treatment of disease by chemical substances.

Chill The condition where the dog's resistance is lowered and infection therefore gains entry to the body. This lowering of resistance is usually associated with cold, damp, exhaustion or under-feeding. Initially the symptoms are only that the dog does not appear fit but, when the infection develops, signs of ill-health become more apparent.

Choking Strictly, this refers to impeded respiration, but many people also use the term to include the obstruction of the pharynx and oesophagus so that food cannot be passed to the stomach.

It usually results from swallowing, or attempting to swallow, bones or large masses of food, but it can be caused by other objects such as pins, needles, wire, fruit-stones, etc. It may also follow infection or inflammation of the throat, oesophagus or bronchi where catarrh is produced.

As a broad generalisation for the owner, the condition can be divided into those cases where the dog's attack occurs suddenly, without warning, and those where a series of increasingly severe attacks develop. The former usually indicates that a foreign body has been swallowed and is causing a blockage, the latter that infec-

Colic

tion, congestion of the lungs or inflammation (qq.v.) is the cause.

To treat the condition, the cause must be discovered. The dog should be examined, the mouth opened and the throat felt for any obstruction. Food and water should be offered only in small amounts and if this is refused or aggravates the choking, it should be immediately taken away. Fresh air helps, while stroking the throat often gives relief.

In any case of choking that does not recover within a few minutes, the advice of a veterinary surgeon must be obtained. A physical examination, possibly including X-rays, is needed, and the heart should be examined.

Chorea (St Vitus's Dance)   The name given to uncontrolled irregular contractions of one or more muscles. Almost any part of the body may be involved, but this condition most commonly affects the muscles of the limbs (perhaps one fore-leg and one hind-leg), or the muscles of the head, shoulder and neck. Occasionally the muscles of the abdomen may contract, in which case the dog may appear to be suffering from hiccoughs.

The most common cause of this condition is damage due to infection of the nerve supply of the relevant muscles. It is often seen as an after-effect of distemper.

Veterinary advice must be obtained.

Claws, Inflamed, *see* Feet, Diseases of.
Cleft Palate, *see* Hereditary Abnormalities.
Coal Gas Poisoning, *see* Poisoning, Carbon Monoxide.
Coccidiosis, *see* Parasites, Internal.
Cod-Liver Oil   An easily obtained source of vitamins A and D. A good dietary supplement, but one that should not be given in excess. A 5 ml teaspoonful once a week is sufficient for the normal dog. It is also supplied in capsules (give 2 per week).

Cod-liver oil should be stored in the cool and away from light.

It can also be used to treat some eye conditons.

Cold Abscess   A term used for an abscess that is slow to come to a 'head' (*see* Abscess).
Cold Nose, *see* Nose.
Colic   Pain in the abdomen caused generally by indigestion, flatulence, constipation or a swallowed foreign body. The condition is common in puppies when they have over-eaten or have been given a change in diet; and in the suckling puppy it may denote that the bitch is not well. Unless a foreign body is present, the

Colitis

attack is usually temporary. Discomfort is felt, the dog whines (or if a puppy, it cries with a loud piercing sound), tends to tap the abdomen with the hind legs, and is restless.

Food and water should be temporarily withheld, and the dog should be kept warm. A teaspoonful to a tablespoonful (5–15 ml) of baby's gripe-water should be given—the amount depending on the size of the dog.

If recovery is not rapid (within 1 hour), a veterinary surgeon should be consulted.

Colitis Inflammation of the colon or large intestine. The condition may be acute or chronic. It arises from specific infection, chills, the presence of foreign bodies, or from habitual constipation, which can lead to this condition by weakening the control of digestion in these parts of the body.

The usual symptom is diarrhoea, sometimes blood-stained, and containing mucus.

Food and water should be withheld until advice is obtained. A teaspoonful (5 ml) of kaolin emulsion in liquid paraffin can be given every 5 hours.

Collapse In this condition, the dog lies semi-conscious, the body feels cold, the membranes are pallid, the eyes are 'glassy', the breathing is slow and deep and the pulse weak. The cause may be shock, heart attack, haemorrhage or stroke (qq.v.).

No attempt must be made to give liquids by mouth while the dog is in a collapsed state. Veterinary advice must be obtained, and in the meantime the dog should be kept warm and quiet.

Coma Complete loss of consciousness, often with heavy breathing and pupils dilated. This condition may result from e.g. injuries to the head, a stroke, heart attack, circulatory failure, gas poisoning. In many illnesses, it is also the last stage before death.

Treatment Ensure that the dog is lying comfortably without constriction to the chest or abdomen. Pull the tongue out as far as possible and provide a good supply of fresh air. Keep warm, using blankets and hot-water bottles as needed. Provide subdued light and quiet surroundings to prevent disturbance as the dog comes out of the attack. Veterinary advice is essential.

Where the dog lies for a considerable time, it is sensible to turn it over every three to four hours to the other side, to aid circulation.

Conjunctivitis, *see* Eye.

Constipation The dog's motions are large, hard, and dry, and

Cryptorchidism

instead of having a regular action, or motion, it may not pass a stool for a number of days.

In the past, a great deal of attention was placed on regular bowel movements, but it is now known that a dog that does not pass a motion for a week is in little danger provided it is otherwise healthy.

Increased exercise, together with food devoid of biscuits, will often cure the condition. Liquid paraffin can be given (5–15 ml depending on the size of the dog). The addition of liver to the diet is also helpful. The feeding of bones must be avoided at all times.

In prolonged cases an enema (q.v.) may be necessary.

Consumption, *see* Tuberculosis.
Contusions, *see* Bruises.
Convulsions in Puppies, *see* Fits.
Coprophagia The eating of stools (*see* Appetite, Depraved).
Corns The dog does not normally suffer from corns.
Cough There are many causes. A short dry cough may occur with pharyngitis. Laryngitis tends to produce a dry, loud, hard cough. Dogs that have been boarded in kennels often return with this type of cough because of excessive barking. Wheezy coughs may result from asthma. In puppies, coughing may be due to worms. A deep cough occurring whenever a dog becomes excited or takes exercise may indicate heart trouble.

Because of the wide range of causes, it is essential to try to determine the cause of a cough as this provides the key to treatment. Veterinary advice is therefore needed for all but a temporary cough.

For home treatment, a child's cough medicine, given as for a child, is often helpful. A mixture of equal amounts of white of egg, honey and water can be given every half-hour (5–15 ml, but as this is a safe treatment the dose is not very important).

Affected dogs should be protected from cold and damp, and not over-exercised.

Cramp This condition is rare in the dog, but it may sometimes occur when it suffers from heart, circulatory or kidney trouble. It is also occasionally seen in racing greyhounds during or just after a race. Warmth, rest and massage, together with an addition of honey and a small amount of salt to the food, are indicated.

Cryptorchidism The condition in the male in which one or both testes do not descend from the abdomen into the scrotum at the usual time. The cause may be hereditary.

Cystitis

A dog with this condition may be unable to reproduce. The skin may be affected because hormonal activity causes thickened skin on the back, sides and legs where hair may not grow and there may be abnormal pigmentation.
See also Monorchid.

Cystitis Inflammation of the bladder. This condition is more common in the bitch than the dog, and may be due to bacterial infection, mechanical irritation due to the presence of stones (calculi), or injury.

Symptoms Frequent urination, but only small amounts of urine passed at each attempt, and that with difficulty. The urine may be blood-stained or highly coloured. Occasionally blood is seen at the end of the urine flow. Pain may be shown if the abdomen is pressed. In acute cases there may be a high temperature, loss of appetite and lethargy.

Treatment must be undertaken by a veterinary surgeon, but the owner should encourage the dog to drink water and ensure that urine is being passed, as if the flow becomes obstructed, the case becomes extremely critical.

Cysts Swellings that contain fluid other than blood or pus.
See also Abscess; Haematoma.

The common form is a retention cyst where a secretory tissue or gland produces a secretion which is unable to escape as the drainage duct is blocked.

INTER-DIGITAL CYSTS These are swellings that appear between the toes, usually caused by a blockage of the sweat glands of the feet. They should be treated by placing the foot in a bowl of warm water to which some salt has been added. This tends to draw the swelling to a head. When it ruptures, it should be cleaned with warm water and salt as described above, three or four times a day. Occasionally the swelling has to be lanced.

It can also be caused by a foreign body, e.g. grass seed, entering the foot.

SEBACEOUS CYSTS These are formed in the skin when the gland that provides 'grease' to a hair becomes blocked. They occur most commonly in elderly dogs. The contents of such cysts is often very thick.

Provided it does not worry the dog, there is no reason to treat this type of cyst. If, however, it causes discomfort, ruptures, or is unsightly, it can be removed surgically.

Debility

RANULA (also called a *salivary cyst*) A swelling seen in the mouth below the tongue, which contains a yellow salivary fluid. It is caused by a blockage of the drainage duct of a salivary gland. Surgery is indicated to correct the condition.

Dandruff (Scurf) A condition of the skin where flakes of dry dead skin are found in the coat. It can result from poor functioning of the sebaceous glands in the skin, or may also be caused by ill-health, lack of exercise or incorrect feeding.

The dog should be groomed twice daily, first with a comb to remove mats and dead hair, then with a stiff brush. The brushing should be carried out vigorously to stimulate the circulation and glands in the skin. The dog should be given plenty of exercise and good food to which a small amount of olive oil (about 5 ml once a week) should be added, as this contains a form of fat that is needed for skin health.

Once a week the dog should be bathed using a dog shampoo; the printed instructions should be followed exactly.

Deafness The inability to hear, which may be partial or complete, which occurs most commonly in old dogs. Deafness may also be a congenital defect in some white dogs.

Causes Malformation, malfunction, or injury to the internal ear, eustachian tube, nervous system, etc. or obstruction of the passage of sound into the ear. A temporary interruption of the passage of sound may result from a collection of wax and other matter that adheres to the surface of the external ear passage.

Treatment Veterinary advice is essential. If the ear is damaged or not functioning properly, it is possible that treatment will not be successful, but when the passage of sound into the ear is merely interrupted, the condition can often be completely cured. If wax, etc., is present, it can be removed by the use of a wax solvent or olive oil. Never force cotton wool into the ear, as this may press the wax further down the passage.

Hair should be cut away from the ear flap if it appears to be blocking the entrance to the ear. Occasionally the entrance to the external ear has to be surgically altered to aid the circulation of air.

Debarking An operation (rarely carried out) to reduce the amount of noise produced by a dog that barks to excess. However, in some cases, it may not prove successful, as the ability to bark may return.

Debility A weakness of the body, or of one or more of the body

Deformities

systems, so that the dog is unable to withstand any strain placed upon it, or in severe cases to carry out the normal body functions.

The condition may occur at any time of life, but is most common in old age.

The cause must be determined. A veterinary surgeon should be consulted. Remedial measures include good food, supplied in small amounts several times a day; a sensible amount of exercise; fresh air; rest; and anything that provides mental interest.

Deformities It is possible for any part of the body to be deformed, either from birth or because of injury or malnutrition. In most cases medical treatment is of doubtful use. Surgery will often correct deformities such as cleft palate, hip dysplasia, etc. *See also* Hereditary Abnormalities.

Delirium A condition where the dog is in a state similar to that of a fit. Symptoms are continuous howling or barking, great excitement and restlessness. It can have a number of causes such as the after-effects of distemper, uraemia, jaundice (in some cases), sunstroke, and allergic reactions.

Veterinary attention is essential. The dog should be kept as quiet as possible until help arrives. Noise and sudden movement by those near the dog should be avoided. Keep the dog cool, but with a good supply of fresh air and restrain it by any method possible if it is tending to injure itself.

Demodectic Mange, *see* Mange.

Dental Fistula, *see* Teeth.

Dentition, *see* Teeth.

Depraved Appetite, *see* Appetite, Depraved.

Dermatitis Strictly, any inflammation of the skin, but the term is commonly used to refer to those inflammatory conditions of the skin where there is also irritation.

Destruction of Dogs Euthanasia should not be carried out except by a person trained in the best methods. For the owner faced with this difficult and unpleasant task without any chance of expert help, the only way is to shoot the dog using a 'humane killer'.

Trained persons use injections, electrical euthanasia or carbon dioxide.

Whenever an inexperienced person has to carry out this procedure it is advisable to give the dog a large dose of tranquilliser or sleeping tablets beforehand.

Diagnosis

No person who is not trained in this procedure should destroy a dog unless this is absolutely unavoidable.

Dew-Claws These are to be found on the inner side of each fore-foot, and sometimes on the hind feet. They have little use, but occasionally assist a dog to turn sharply when running.

They are often removed when a puppy is 3 to 5 days old.

REMOVAL They should be cut off close to the limb with a sharp pair of scissors. Bleeding should be controlled by placing permanganate of potash crystals or Friar's Balsam on the cut. If bleeding persists, the wound should be bandaged for a few minutes.

If for any reason these claws have to be removed when a dog is over 1 week old, a local or general anaesthetic must be used and this operation must be carried out by a veterinary surgeon.

Dewlap A mass of skin hanging on the lower part of the neck under the chin and throat. Most commonly seen in certain breeds, e.g. Bloodhound.

Diabetes Insipidus A condition where the dog produces a large amount of very dilute watery urine. It is caused by an alteration in the amount of vasopressin produced by the hypothalamus. Veterinary treatment is essential.

Diabetes Mellitus A condition where carbohydrate is not properly digested and utilised within the body, as insufficient insulin is being produced in the pancreas. Usually there is a high blood sugar level and sugar is found in the urine. Blood and urine tests confirm the diagnosis.

A dog suffering from this condition tends to eat excessively, lose weight, pass urine that tends to leave a white deposit when dried, and drinks excessively.

Treatment, which includes careful feeding, tablets, injections of insulin, and massive doses of vitamin C, must be carried out on veterinary advice.

Diabetic dogs have a shortened expectation of life.

It must be stressed that if a dog is receiving daily injections for this condition, the diet (*see* Section 3) must be regulated, both in amount and content, while exercise must also be controlled.

In the advanced stage it is sometimes found that the dog's breath smells of acetone—a smell identical to nail-varnish remover. Cataracts may develop on the lens of the eye (*see* Eye).

See also Pseudo Diabetes.

Diagnosis The opinion, based on scientific knowledge and good clinical observation, formed as to the cause and nature of ill-health. Training in the art and science of medicine is essential. Diagnostic aids (such as blood tests and urine samples, to name two of a vast number) help the clinician to reach his opinion.

Diaphragmatic Rupture, *see* Hernia.

Diarrhoea A condition where the fluid content of the stools is greatly increased. Associated symptoms are thirst, loss of appetite and frequent rectal straining. Sometimes mucus is present in the stools.

Causes Lowered resistance, infection, parasitic infestation, mental upsets, or irritation due to ingested abnormal substances or poisons.

Treatment Give no water or food for 24 hours. A 5 ml teaspoonful of kaolin and liquid paraffin emulsion may be given three times a day.

Where diarrhoea is acute, the dog is obviously ill; if recovery does not occur within two days, the advice of a veterinary surgeon is needed.

Recent research has shown that Alsatians may have an inherited tendency to chronic diarrhoea.

IN PUPPIES Changes of diet, unclean conditions, worms, or the ill-health of the dam may be causes.

The cause must be found and remedied; the puppy should be kept warm and given a few (3 to 5) drops of baby's gripe-water. Where the bitch is ill, it may be necessary to hand-feed the puppies for a few days.

Dislocations Injuries to joints where the bones concerned do not make a proper connection. Often there is bruising of the surrounding tissue, and the ligaments holding the joint together may be damaged. Dislocations are usually caused by mechanical stress or accidents.

The dog frequently will show no sign of pain, but will not use the affected limb. The joint may appear to be distorted. The animal should be kept as quiet as possible until veterinary advice has been obtained.

The diagnosis should be confirmed by X-ray examination and other investigatory procedures to determine the amount of injury.

Treatment aims to reduce (reposition) the dislocation, usually under a general anaesthetic. After the operation, the joint may have to be immobilised.

Distemper

Distemper A virus infection that affects dogs, wolves, foxes, stoats, ferrets and mink. It cannot infect humans or cats. The disease is often fatal; mortality may often be as high as 80 per cent.
Symptoms If it has no other complicating infections, the dog appears unwell, has a high temperature and is off its food. Within a few days, it recovers. However, in most cases, complications do occur because other infections enter the body, and damage to the nervous system may follow.

The normal case of distemper shows signs of infection in various ways. There may be diarrhoea, eye discharges, a greeny-yellow nasal discharge or a cough. Where the virus damages the nervous system, signs of unco-ordination, muscle twitches or fits may occur.
Treatment Once the virus has attacked the dog, veterinary treatment is difficult, but should be started as soon as possible. Antiserum, antibiotics and symptomatic treatment are required. Recovery cannot be guaranteed.

It is far better to try to prevent the disease than to treat it; *see* Prevention; *see also* Hard-Pad Disease.

PREVENTION Dogs can be protected against distemper by the use of vaccines. However, new-born puppies whose dam is protected against this disease receive protection from the first milk that they obtain. This milk contains immune antibodies and provides a 'natural' resistance (colostral immunity) to infection for a period (usually until 8 to 12 weeks of age). It must be stressed that this type of protection can occur only when the bitch herself is protected against this disease.

Protection against distemper, given artificially by injection to older dogs, lasts for a variable period, usually about 2 years. It is therefore necessary to boost such protection at regular intervals. A vaccine will not stimulate immunity in a dog that is already resistant to the disease.

Both distemper and measles are caused by myxo-viruses. A modified virus of measles is therefore sometimes used to confer protection to a dog against distemper—it has the advantage that it can be given while colostral immunity still exists and also that resistance to distemper develops rapidly.

The normal vaccines take some time to become effective. Where protection is required almost immediately, temporary resistance can be given by the injection of immune serum or concentrated immune serum.

Distemper Teeth

All these injections must be given by a veterinary surgeon.

In many instances the distemper vaccine is combined with vaccines against other diseases (e.g. viral hepatitis, leptospirosis). Usually it is necessary to give two injections, approximately 2 weeks apart, when such combined vaccines are used.

Distemper Teeth Teeth of which the enamel is damaged during the period of tooth formation. Originally the condition was given this name as those puppies that recovered from distemper usually showed damage to the dental enamel. The enamel is not properly deposited on the surface of the dentine as the teeth develop, and yellow or brown pitted areas can be seen on the tooth surfaces.

Distension of Abdomen, *see* Dropsy; Flatulence.

Docking, *see* Tail.

Doses All drugs must be used with care. The dose must be accurately assessed and carefully given. This dosage is calculated from the size, weight, age and condition of the dog. Not only must the right amount be supplied but it must be given at the correct time.

Drugs of all types must be treated with respect.

Dosing, *see* Section 4.

Dropsy (Ascites, Abdominal Dropsy) Although dropsy can mean the accumulation of fluid under the skin, the term is most commonly used for the condition where there is an accumulation of fluid within the abdominal cavity. This fluid is usually yellow straw-coloured.

The condition must not be confused with peritonitis (where there is infection or inflammation); distended bladder; urine in the abdominal cavity from a ruptured bladder (here the dog is extremely ill and death follows rapidly if the condition is not surgically corrected); or pregnancy.

Cause Usually heart, circulatory, liver or kidney disturbance.

Symptoms Enlargement of the abdomen not restricted to any one part. Breathing is usually distressed.

Treatment Depends on the cause but must be undertaken by a veterinary surgeon.

Drowning Death by drowning is directly due to asphyxia, since the air in the lungs and bronchi is replaced by water and the animal's blood cannot therefore be re-oxygenated.

If, when the dog is discovered, the heart is still beating, artificial respiration (q.v.) should be attempted.

Dysentery A condition in which blood is released into the intestine. This blood is passed from the bowels, with or without diarrhoea. Mucus is usually present.

Veterinary advice must be obtained. Food and water should be withheld for the time being. Warmth is essential.

Dyspepsia This term refers to digestive difficulty and is often used as a synonym for indigestion. It should, however, include all conditions that cause pain or discomfort within the digestive system.

EAR (*see also* Deafness)

Ear-Ache

Symptoms Head shaking. The head is often held downwards and to one side. The dog does not like having the ear touched; it may be quiet, and avoids noise and humans.

Treatment Examine the dog to see whether there is matted hair or wax in the external part of the ear. Look for foreign bodies (such as a grass seed), an abscess, growths and abnormalities of any kind.

A few drops of warmed olive oil put into the ear often give relief. However, unless recovery is very rapid, veterinary advice is required.

Canker A vague term applied to conditions of the external ear where exudate collects on the visible part of the ear. Canker is usually associated with ulceration.

The cause is usually lack of air to that part of the ear external to the ear drum. This is in turn caused by excessive hair in the ear, misshaped ear 'flaps', dirt, or swelling from other causes. This lack of air produces conditions where inflammation and often infection can develop. The exudate so produced tends to dry and accumulate and so further restricts the supply of air. The condition is most commonly seen in those breeds with long pendulous ear flaps, e.g. Spaniels.

The dog suffering from this condition tends to shake its head and scratch at the ears. Often the ear most severely affected is held downwards. The ear itself often feels hot, appears tender and inflamed, has a brown discharge and may smell offensively.

It is wrong to try to treat this condition with cotton wool probes as, although some of the discharge will be removed, the remainder is forced further down the external ear passage.

The ear should be gently cleaned with a solution of a teaspoonful of bicarbonate of soda to 100 ml of warm water or with warm olive oil. Alternatively a wax solvent can be obtained. Any hair that is obstructing the flow of air should be removed. The dog should be kept away from heat while under treatment. If a quick response is not obtained, veterinary attention is essential.

Hydrogen peroxide or methylated spirit should not be used.

See also Ear-Ache.

Cropping   The reshaping of the ear flap by surgical amputation of part of the flap. The procedure is prohibited in many countries, including the British Isles, as inhumane.

In the United States of America, dogs of the following breeds may be so altered: Bouvier des Flandres, Boxer, Briard, Doberman Pinscher, Schnauzer, Great Dane, Manchester Terrier, Affenpinscher, Griffon Bruxellois, Miniature Pinscher and Boston Terrier.

Discharge from, *see* Canker.

Growths in   These can be of many types, the commonest being polypi, warts, or granulation tissue formed because of irritation of some kind. Growths that rub against each other may become ulcerated, with an ensuing infection, and an unpleasant-smelling discharge results.

Treatment must be by a veterinary surgeon and often involves the surgical removal of the growths under a general anaesthetic.

Hairlessness of   This condition is usually caused by the dog rubbing its ear because of some form of irritation, infection, or a hormonal imbalance.

The cause must be determined and treated. Olive oil massaged into the skin may help.

Inflammation   An inflamed ear is hot, tender when touched, and with some swelling. The dog holds the affected ear downwards, and the irritation tends to make it rub and scratch. This condition is seen most commonly in long-eared dogs.

Wherever possible, the cause must be determined. If the inflammation is due to dirt or a scratch the ear should be cleaned with olive oil and then dressed with acriflavine emulsion. If the cause is parasitic, because of an infection with ear mites (which can usually be seen in the wax of the ear under a hand lens), the ear should be treated twice weekly with benzyl benzoate emulsion, as follows: a few drops of the liquid are put into the ear, which is then gently massaged to work the emulsion over all the surfaces. The dog should then be allowed to shake the excess out of the ear.

Eclampsia

Other causes of inflammation include wax, dirt, insects, water or foreign bodies.
See also Grass Seeds.
Scurfiness of May be caused by parasites (q.v.).
See also Dandruff.
Swelling on Flap of, *see* Haematoma.
Ulceration, *see* Canker.
Wounds Dogs often receive injuries to the edge of the ear flap. These may bleed profusely and, although not serious, can be very difficult to heal as the dog scratches and shakes its head because of the irritation, and this prevents healing.

The actual cut should be cleaned and dressed with a soothing lotion; acriflavine emulsion is ideal. A pad of cotton wool should be placed on the head, and the ear flap laid back onto this. Another pad is then placed on the ear and the whole head bandaged to ensure that both the ear and the dressing stay in place. This bandage should be firm, but not so tight that it restricts breathing. It should be possible to insert two fingers under the bandage at the underside of the neck. To keep the bandage in place, stick adhesive tape over it and also over the skin for 2 cm each side of the area covered by the bandage.

This should be left in place for a week unless it becomes disarranged by the dog or signs of infection occur—these are demonstrated by the dog becoming unwell or an unpleasant smell developing.

Eclampsia A fit-like attack where the body reacts violently to any stimulus. It occurs occasionally in dogs of either sex (especially in Poodles), and especially in the nursing bitch.

The condition is caused by a shortage of available calcium in the blood. This does not mean that the dog has received insufficient calcium in its diet, or that it has not enough calcium within its body, but that it cannot transport calcium from the body reserves into the blood-stream quickly enough when a sudden demand occurs.

The dog should be kept quiet, away from noise or bright light, and offered milk if it will drink. Sedatives may reduce the symptoms. Immediate response is obtained if calcium is supplied, preferably by injection. Veterinary advice is required.

Where a bitch is feeding puppies and is affected by this condition, it is advisable to remove these for a few hours and also to

Ectropion

supplement their feeding if possible (*see* Hand-Rearing of Puppies).
Ectropion, *see* Eyelid, Everted.
Eczema   A non-contagious skin disease which is very common in dogs. The skin becomes inflamed and infection may subsequently develop. Sores, rashes, and moist areas are common. Most visible signs are produced through the dog scratching and biting at the inflamed areas.
Symptoms   Skin irritation; the dog scratching, licking and biting itself. Clusters of fine vesicles appear at different parts, the skin afterwards becoming dry and scaly unless the dog by constant licking makes the areas sore and raw. Areas principally attacked are around the eyes, the lips, outside and inside the ears, along the top of the back, and the root of the tail; but any part may become affected.
Causes   These are not fully understood. They may be fungi, allergy, flea-bite allergy, over-dosing with vitamins, vitamin deficiency, lack of certain types of fat in the diet, hormonal imbalance, sensitivity to strong light or excessive bathing.
Treatment   As there are so many different possible causes, the owner should consult a veterinary surgeon, who should be supplied with as full a past history of the dog as possible. Laboratory tests are often used to determine the cause.

For home treatment, it is essential to start by examining the dog for signs of external parasites (q.v.). If these are present, bath the dog with an anti-parasite shampoo, following the directions carefully.

Moist sores should be gently cleaned to remove hair or dirt that is stuck to the area and then powdered with a wound dressing powder or dabbed with calamine lotion. Once dry, they should be treated as dry sores.

Dry sores should be covered with a thin layer of acriflavine emulsion, baby oil or zinc and caster oil.

The aim is to dry a moist sore and to prevent a dry sore from becoming too hard.

At all times the dog should be kept cool, given plenty of exercise, and prevented, as far as possible, from licking (q.v.), scratching or biting the affected areas. Gentle grooming helps, and so does the addition of a small amount (about 1 cc) of margarine or vegetable oil to the diet once a week.
Elbow, Capped, *see* Bursitis.

Emphysema

Elongated Soft Palate, *see* Hereditary Abnormalities.

Emaciation Loss of condition, with debility and wasting. The mouth and conjunctival membranes often appear pale. Strictly this is a condition caused by starvation, but in general use the term is applied to the condition whatever the cause; it therefore includes abnormal conditions affecting the health of the body where loss of weight occurs.

Causes These are numerous and diverse: e.g. infection, malignant tumours, parasitism, nephritis, diabetes, senility (qq.v.). The cause must be determined before treatment can be properly carried out.

As a home measure, one should treat for worms if these are present. Food should be supplied in small quantities at frequent intervals, and should be very nourishing. Vitamin and mineral supplements should be added to the diet. Tonics are useful. However, it must be stressed that treatment should be carried out under the guidance of a veterinary surgeon.

Emesis The act of expelling the stomach contents via the mouth. Dogs may eat grass to give bulk within the stomach so that they can vomit.

See also Travel Sickness; Vomiting.

Emetics Drugs or other agents that cause vomiting. They are used to expel from the stomach harmful substances that have been ingested.

An effective home emetic is a crystal of **washing** soda about 1 to 2 cm in diameter—the dog is made to swallow this, and vomiting usually follows in about 30 seconds. For a very small dog, a crystal about 0·5 cm in diameter is sufficient.

Note—Take care not to give caustic soda by mistake.

Emphysema The abnormal presence of air in a part of the body, usually the lungs. Can be separated into two types: that which affects the lungs, and that which occurs in other parts of the body.

PULMONARY EMPHYSEMA: ACUTE Associated with broncho-pneumonia or a condition where the trachea is partially obstructed. It may start suddenly, and may be associated with a heart condition, especially in the older dog.

A persistent cough, difficult respiration and discomfort are the usual symptoms.

PULMONARY EMPHYSEMA: CHRONIC Associated with chronic bronchitis usually due to poor circulation. The symptoms are

Encephalitis

difficulty in respiration, and coughing when the dog moves from a warm atmosphere to a cold, or when exercised.

The distinction between acute and chronic pulmonary emphysema is not easy to make. Veterinary treatment is essential. A warm atmosphere and restricted exercise helps the patient. An inhalant, such as Friar's Balsam in hot water, may give relief.

SUBCUTANEOUS EMPHYSEMA   Not very frequently seen. It can be caused by an infected wound where the infection produces gas or when air enters the wound. The area is swollen. It may be possible for the hand to feel the movement of the air within the tissues, and a 'crackling' noise may be heard.

Treatment   Requires veterinary advice. The original wound should be opened to aid the dispersal of infection and gas. Hot fomentations help this dispersal. Antibiotics are essential. The dog should be kept warm and quiet.

Encephalitis   Inflammation of the brain (*see* Brain, Inflammation of).

Enema   The injection of a fluid into the rectum via the anus. Enemas are used to relieve constipation and occasionally as a means of supplying nutrient, salts or fluid to a sick dog.

The procedure can be used to treat worm infestation.

Enteritis, *see* Bowel, Inflammation of.

Enterotomy   An operation to open the intestine, which is later sutured to seal this incision. It is usually performed where there is an obstruction of the intestine, e.g. by a foreign body.

In an enterectomy operation, a portion of the bowel itself is removed.

Entropion, *see* Eyelid, Inverted.

Epilepsy   A chronic nervous disorder where there is sudden loss of consciousness usually with muscular convulsions. It is associated with a disorder of part of the brain. A dog which has suffered from one attack is likely to undergo further attacks.

Causes   Post-distemper encephalitis, brain damage through injury, inflammatory changes due to infection, tumours, local biological changes such as blood-glucose and blood-gas levels, hormonal disturbances, fatigue, dietary deficiencies, worm infestation and even emotional stress. Congenital defects and hereditary predisposition may also be involved.

Treatment   Can be divided into two parts: the removal of the cause (if possible), and the symptomatical treatment.

Eye

The removal of parasites, and the correction of haematological abnormalities, where these exist, bring relief. Otherwise the symptoms must be controlled. Anticonvulsant drugs are of help, but act so as to mask the trouble rather than cure it. It is essential that owners follow the instructions of their veterinary adviser even though the dog appears to be cured. Drugs must be given at definite times; if they are administered irregularly, the dog's chance of recovery is greatly reduced.

It is essential that this condition is treated by a veterinary surgeon.

Epistaxis Bleeding from the nose (*see* Haemorrhage, Nasal).

Epulis, *see* Gum, Growth on.

Erythema A red and inflamed condition of the skin, the redness temporarily disappearing on pressure. Seen mainly on the inside of the ear flaps, inside the thighs and fore-legs. There is often much irritation, so that the dog licks and scratches the affected areas.

Treat as for eczema (q.v.).

Euthanasia, *see* Destruction of Dogs.

Exhaustion (due to over-exertion) The dog is very languid, breathes heavily, and has a fast but weak pulse.

Treatment Rest is essential. It is sensible to give ¼ to 1 teaspoonful of brandy (depending on the size of the dog) in a little water, and to restrict food for a few hours. Supply honey if the dog is very weak.

EYE (*see also* Blindness).

Blue Eye The term usually used for *Keratitis profunda*, which is a condition associated with, or following, infection with canine virus hepatitis. It affects one or both eyes and is sudden in onset.

The affected eye is not painful and does not shed tears, but becomes a dense diffuse blue in appearance. This condition usually disappears in 7 to 10 days without treatment, although chloramphenicol eye ointment should be used three times a day to try to prevent infection entering the altered tissues.

Occasionally, where one eye is affected, the second eye may show this condition after the first has cleared.

Blue eye is also very occasionally seen in a dog that has been given an injection of live viral hepatitis vaccine.

See also Blue Film over.

Blue Film over This condition, common in dogs, may be due to a variety of causes. Most often it results from injury, infection

Eye

or reaction to drugs, chemicals or vaccines. It can also be caused by dust, foreign bodies or gases, or it may be secondary to other eye conditions.

Veterinary treatment is essential, as the cause must be identified. Bathing with a weak solution of warm boracic lotion may ease the discomfort, while a drop of cod-liver oil on the eye may assist in many cases.

It is essential that the dog be prevented from rubbing or otherwise damaging the eye.

See also Blue Eye.

Cataract A pathological change in the lens of the eye or its capsule which diminishes its transparency. It does not cause pain. There is a disturbance of vision according to the amount of opacity present.

Causes Injury; hereditary; diseases of the eye which interfere with the nutrition of the lens; diabetes mellitus; senility.

Symptoms The formation of an opaque spot or patch on the lens. When it occurs in young dogs, the whole lens is often involved, but in the old dog it generally starts as a small speck which gradually increases in size. The cornea, or front of the eye, generally remains clear. There is loss of vision of the affected eye to a greater or lesser extent, according to the size and density of the cataract.

Treatment Eye drops and drugs rarely have much effect. The surgical removal of the lens is often very effective in increasing the ability of the dog to see. However, this operation is not always successful, as other conditions of the eye may prevent improvement. Eye surgery of this sort is acceptable in the dog.

Older dogs may suffer from 'senile cataract', where there is a change of colour of the lens, but the dog's vision is not affected.

Conjunctivitis (sore or weak eyes) Inflammation of the conjunctival membrane lining the inside of the eyelids, which becomes congested and dark red in colour. There is a watery discharge which tends to become brown, yellow or white if infection is present. It may collect round the eye and form crusts, and, if it continues for a period, may cause sores round the eyelids and loss of hair in that region.

Treatment In simple cases, an application of boracic lotion made by dissolving half a teaspoonful of boracic acid crystals in 0.15 litres of boiled water is often sufficient to cure the condition. This should be applied every two hours.

Eye

Soothing eye ointment is also helpful. However, as with all inflammations or infections, veterinary advice is advisable.

It is essential to keep the eye clean and to prevent the dog from rubbing it. Self injury, however, is sometimes difficult to prevent.

Discharge from This discharge may be watery or purulent. It may start as a clean watery liquid and then change in composition to a yellow, grey or black mucus. If one eye only is affected, it is safe to assume that there is no general constitutional upset and that the cause is probably localised. Infections such as distemper (q.v.) often produce an associated brown mucus or a green or yellow purulent eye discharge.

Infection must be treated. The eye should be thoroughly examined to ensure that no foreign body is present. They should be bathed with warm water to remove discharges and then treated with warm boracic lotion. This cleansing should be carried out as often as needed to ensure that the eyes are kept clean. Neglect of this precaution can lead to ulceration developing round the eyes.

Neglected eyes soon develop additional troubles, so it is always advisable to obtain professional advice.

Dislocation of This condition is usually seen in breeds with prominent eyes, such as the Pug, Pekinese, King Charles Spaniel, etc. It is commonly caused by fighting or by a blow to the head at the side or back of the eye.

The eye is forced forward, and the eyelid passes under it into the cavity behind, preventing the return of the eye to the proper position.

Immediate treatment is essential. If at all possible this should be carried out by a veterinary surgeon, so that the dog may have the best chance of recovery.

The eye and eyelids are bathed with a lubricant (for home attention, cod-liver oil can be used), and the eyelids are worked away from the eye until the eye returns to its proper position.

The danger of this condition is that as soon as the eye becomes dislocated it begins to swell. The larger it becomes, the harder is the task of replacement. When the eye has been displaced for several hours, it is often found that vision has been lost.

A veterinary surgeon will often replace the eye and then suture the eyelids together for a few days, to ensure that the eye stays in place.

Eyelashes, Ingrowing

Dropsy of, *see* Glaucoma.
Foreign Bodies in Occasionally objects such as hay, grass seeds, grit, etc. become lodged under an eyelid.

Because of the intense irritation, the dog rubs the eye, causing a profuse discharge, and sores on the skin near the eye.

Treatment by a veterinary surgeon is required as it is usually necessary to anaesthetise the eye, or even the dog, before the foreign body can be removed. An examination is also required in order to determine whether damage has been caused to the surface of the eye.
Glaucoma A condition of the eye where the amount of fluid within the eye increases. The eye becomes enlarged and the visible surface assumes a blue-white colour. It is usually associated with an alteration of the normal drainage of the eye.

Veterinary treatment for this condition is essential.
Keratitis Inflammation of the cornea, usually associated with conjunctivitis, which may be due to injury or a foreign body rubbing on the surface of the eye. The cornea appears opaque. Ulceration of this area may also exist. It is unwise for treatment to be given except on veterinary advice. As a first aid treatment, a drop of cod-liver oil can be put onto the eye.
Progressive Retinal Atrophy, *see* Hereditary Abnormalities.
Squint This incorrect positioning of one eye in relation to the other. This condition is relatively rare in the dog. If it is decided to correct the squint, surgery will be required.
Ulceration of Usually the result of injury to the surface of the eye. Veterinary attention is essential. As a first aid measure, a drop of cod-liver oil may be put onto the eye.

Eyelashes, Ingrowing Technically known as trichiasis. Hairs become misplaced so that they touch the eye, usually because the eyelid is mis-shaped.

There is usually watering from the eye, in some cases pain and fear of bright light. Inflammation, ulceration, and acute pain can result.

Correction is achieved by removal of the hairs or by an operation.
EYELID
Blepharitis Inflammation of the eyelids, which may be due to irritation or to an infection. The caked discharges must be softened and removed by bathing with warm boracic solution; the

Eyelid

area should be dried with cotton wool or a clean white cloth, and the eye then dressed with a soothing eye ointment (such as golden eye ointment). Where infection is present, an antibiotic eye ointment is required, so a veterinary surgeon should be consulted. Cod-liver oil is of value when applied locally for some conditions of inflammation of the eyelids.

Ectropion, *see* Eyelid, Everted.
Entropion, *see* Eyelid, Inverted.
Everted   Known as ectropion. It is seen as normal in some breeds, e.g. St Bernard, Bloodhound, but it may occur in any breed.

The lower lid falls away from the eye, to show the red conjunctiva. Where necessary the condition can be corrected by an operation.

Inverted   Known as entropion. The eyelids tend to turn in onto the eye, and the condition is usually noticed because of the watery discharge produced by the rubbing of the hairs on the eye itself. This condition can be corrected by surgical methods, while soothing eye ointments or lotions give relief where irritation exists.

Sore Eyelid   The membrane of the eye and surrounding area appear red and inflamed. There is a discharge, and the dog tends to rub the eye, so that the surrounding skin becomes swollen, inflamed and raw.

The eye should be cleaned with warm water and treated with boracic solution every few hours. Recovery should be quick. If it is not, veterinary attention is essential.

Stye   A small hard swelling on the edge of the eyelid, which may occur without any other symptom or be associated with other infections or disease.

Veterinary treatment is advisable. The stye may be caused by infection at the base of an eyelash, in which case the extraction of the eyelash concerned will often correct the condition. The eye should be bathed with an eye lotion and all encrustations removed.

General health should be considered. This is one of the few occasions where a dose of Epsom salts is of use—about $\frac{1}{3}$ to 1 teaspoonful (depending on the size of the dog) in a little water.

Third Eyelid   Dogs have three eyelids, the third being known as the nictitating membrane. It is situated towards the inner canthus (corner) of the eye.

GROWTH ON   This can be mistaken for a growth on the eye. It is in fact a swelling of the Harderian gland, which may be seen as a yellow or red swelling near the inner corner of the eye.

Fading Puppies

PROTRUSION OF   The third eyelid may protrude over the eyeball, causing discomfort and looking unsightly.

This protrusion can occur when the dog is unwell, disappearing when it has recovered. However, in some instances, the membrane remains over the eye, in which case surgery is probably indicated.

Fading Puppies   This term is used when puppies die suddenly during the first week of life, usually without any visible cause. It may be a serious problem for dog breeders. The term was originally used for any death in puppies, but is now restricted to conditions where a puppy cannot maintain its own body temperature due to some factor which so reduces the puppies' resistance that survival is impossible. Usually more than one puppy of a litter is affected.

The causes are numerous, and not all known. Lack of heat, infection, illness of the bitch, and the inability of the pup to obtain enough nourishment have all been implicated.

Puppies must be kept warm and the bitch contented. Care must be taken to ensure that puppies cannot become separated from the mother. Where one is rejected by her (and this may occur if it is not strong), heat must be supplied to maintain its body temperature. It may be found that the bitch will again accept and care for the puppy, once it is thoroughly warmed.

Whenever this problem occurs, it is essential to obtain veterinary advice in an attempt to determine the cause.

Fainting   Loss of consciousness (*see* Heart Attack; Shock; Stroke).

False Heat   A condition where a bitch comes into season at an unexpected time, or where the heat (season) occurs without visible signs. Provided the bitch is not unwell, the condition is usually not serious. However, it is sensible to record the date it starts, as this may help a veterinary surgeon later if the bitch subsequently becomes unwell.

False Pregnancy   This condition can appear in a bitch 3 to 12 weeks after a season if she is not pregnant. It is not necessary for her to have been mated unsuccessfully for this to occur.

The bitch begins to behave as though she was pregnant: she may produce milk, make a bed in preparation for her puppies, may put on weight and become slower in her movements.

Where a bitch has once behaved thus, it is frequently found

Feet, Diseases of

that she will have a false pregnancy after each subsequent season. Allowing her to have a litter of puppies does not prevent a recurrence of false pregnancies after later seasons.

The condition usually will resolve itself after several weeks. However, the bitch is unhappy, and causes the owner to worry. For this reason it is essential that she should have treatment. For home treatment it is necessary to provide increased exercise, a cool bed without too much bedding and a reduction (slight) in the amount of food and water. A 300 mg potassium bromide tablet given twice daily often helps. Where the attack is severe, veterinary attention should be obtained.

Favus A form of ringworm (q.v.).

FEET, DISEASES OF

Cracked or Sore Pads The pads become very dry and brittle, and comparatively large and deep fissures may appear. The feet become very tender and the dog is lame. A small amount of Friar's Balsam placed in the cracks often helps the condition. In very severe cases, the foot should be dressed with acriflavine emulsion, bandaged lightly and enclosed in a child's white sock. The sock should be tied in place by a cord put round the leg above a joint. The sock should not be able to slip down, but the cord should not be so tight as to affect the circulation.

Causes Very commonly extensive exercise over hard and hot surfaces, e.g. roads in hot weather; also running over fields where there is stubble; some infections and diseases such as distemper or hard pad.

If the dog does not recover quickly, veterinary advice is needed.

Eczema A frequent condition which is caused by irritation, so that the dog chews the foot and becomes lame.

Home treatment is to place the foot in a shallow pan containing a weak solution of potassium permanganate for three or four minutes a day. Alternatively a 5 per cent solution of alum can be used. *See also* Eczema.

Foreign Bodies These are not always easy to detect. Some can be discovered only by using an X-ray. Surgery under anaesthetic may be required for their removal.

See also Grass Seeds.

Hard Pads These can be caused by over-exercise on hard or hot surfaces, and can also be seen as one of the end stages of hard pad disease (q.v.).

Feet, Diseases of

Interdigital Cysts, *see* Cysts.
Nails, Inflamed These are usually caused by infection or damage. It is not uncommon for nails to be caught in a crack in a pavement, etc., and become torn. There is swelling, redness, and tenderness at the base of the nail. To treat the condition, soak the foot in a warm antiseptic solution for as long as possible, dry, and powder with any form of talcum powder. Healing is often slow.

Where recovery does not take place quickly, if the condition increases or the dog is unwell, veterinary attention should be obtained.

Nails, Over-Long These can result from lack of exercise, exercise on soft ground or improper positioning of the foot so that the nail does not meet the ground in the normal way. They occur when the nail grows faster than it is worn away, and is also seen where dew-claws are not cut.
Treatment Either exercise on hard surfaces (where this is lacking) or cutting the nails.

If the nail end has entered the tissues, a sore is left after cutting. This should be soaked in a warm salt solution (a 5 ml teaspoonful in 0·5 litre of water).
Toes Broken or Dislocated This can occur in any dog but is most commonly seen in racing Greyhounds.
Treatment Rest, encasing in plaster, occasionally amputation is needed. Veterinary advice is essential.

Fever A condition of the body characterised by an increase of temperature, shivering, lassitude, and loss of appetite.
See also Septicaemia.
Fighting, *see* Section 2, 'Canine Behaviour Patterns'.
Fits These occur when the nervous system of the body is seriously upset, and are usually associated with damage to the brain. They can also occur where the water, salt or hormonal balance is disturbed. Teething and worm infestation in puppies may also produce similar attacks. Veterinary treatment is essential.

As a first aid measure, the dog should be placed in a cool, darkened room and kept quiet. Noise, bright lights or movement by any other thing or person in the room may stimulate the dog. This is to be avoided. Food and water should be withheld during

the attack, and afterwards only a little should be given. Sedatives in small amounts may be given e.g. 300 mg potassium bromide.
See also Eclampsia; Epilepsy.

Flatulence The undue collection of gases in the stomach and intestines. It is seen most commonly in puppies, and is usually caused by a disturbed digestion if abnormal or excessive food has been given, or the dog's digestive process has been upset.

The dog is uncomfortable and restless, and usually has a distended stomach. Pain may follow. There may be vomiting and diarrhoea (qq.v.).

Rest and warmth are essential. Food should be withheld for a while. Water should be restricted. A teaspoonful (5 ml) of baby's gripe-water or, alternatively, a teaspoonful of bicarbonate of soda in a little water can be given.

Recovery should be rapid. If the condition continues for longer than 6 hours, or if the condition of the dog begins to deteriorate, a veterinary surgeon should be consulted.

Fleas Parasitic insects with a complex life-cycle, going through the various stages of egg, larva, and pupa to perfect insect. The eggs are laid on the dog's body and in bedding, between floorboards, etc. From these eventually small grey-white maggots emerge which as a rule assume the pupal stage in a cocoon after about 2 weeks. After a further fortnight the flea itself appears, and the life-cycle recommences. The flea moves by jumping and running. It sucks the dog's blood and is entirely parasitic.

It is usually easy to determine if a dog is suffering from an attack of fleas as these can be seen in the coat. But, where the attack is slight, it may be difficult to find the insects themselves; however, the droppings they produce can be seen. These look like shiny coal dust; if combed out onto wet paper they stain the paper with small brown stains.

Treatment consists of baths with a suitable shampoo or powdering the dog with a dog flea powder specifically made for this problem. There are also safe sprays and insecticidal blocks and similar preparations which can be used in buildings and rooms. The directions must always be accurately followed. It is essential to remember that, because of the parasite's life-cycle, treatment must be continued for several weeks, usually at 4-day intervals, but depending on the treatment used.

Fly Attacks

Bedding should be destroyed or boiled. It is usually not practical to remove floorboards, etc. so the dog has to be treated until all chance of reinfestation has passed.

Fly Attacks These can occur where a wound is left untreated, or when a dog becomes soiled and the excreta is not removed.

The area should be cleaned, hair, fly's eggs and maggots removed if necessary and the skin dried. Talcum powder should be applied.

If the fly maggots have penetrated deeply, a veterinary surgeon should be consulted.

This condition only occurs in dogs that are not properly groomed and cleaned.

Foetal Rickets, *see* Achondroplasia.

Fomentation The treatment of local parts of the body by warm or hot moist applications. Cloths may be wrung out in hot water and laid over the part to be so treated, or the part may be sprayed or soaked. To be effective, the process should be continued for some time, i.e. for at least 5 minutes.

Used for the 'bringing to a head' of an abscess, the treatment of painful bruises, sores, etc.

Foods and Feeding, *see* Section 2, 'Canine Nutrition' and 'Feeding a dog'.

Foot Injuries, *see* Feet, Diseases of; Fractures; Wounds.

Foreign Bodies Swallowed These may be stones, bones, sticks, coins, stockings, etc. It is possible for almost anything to be ingested by an unfortunate dog.

They can become 'stuck' in any part of the digestive tract. This obstruction may be temporary or permanent. In the latter case, surgical removal may be required.

This condition should never be treated without veterinary assistance, but where there is a danger to the dog's life, it must have instant help. A situation of such urgency usually occurs when a foreign body becomes lodged in the dog's throat and prevents it from breathing. The obstruction must be removed at once. With the fingers, or a pair of forceps, the foreign body should be grasped and moved from side to side until it becomes loose. Once it is removed, the dog will normally start to breathe; if not, artificial respiration (q.v.) should be carried out.

See also Bowel, Foreign Bodies in.

Foster Mother A bitch in milk that is used to rear puppies of

Fractures

another bitch who is unable to nurse her own young. If such a bitch is available, this is an ideal way of rearing puppies where their dam cannot do this. But it has the disadvantage that the puppies may not receive maternal antibodies (*see* Immunity).

Fractures Although a dog can readily fracture any bone in its body, it is usually those of the limbs which break. Diagnosis is confirmed by X-rays.

The symptoms of a fracture are deformity, pain and swelling at the seat of fracture, with crepitus (grating together) of the broken ends of the bones when the parts are moved. Where a limb is affected, it is unable to support the dog's weight fully.

There are three kinds of fracture. *Simple,* when one or more bones are broken into two pieces, for example when the two bones of the fore-leg (the radius and ulna) have one break without serious injury to the skin. *Compound,* when in addition to the fracture, the skin and other tissues are torn exposing the bone. *Comminuted,* when the bone is broken into several pieces. It is, of course, possible to have a compound comminuted fracture.

There is a 'false form' of fracture that occasionally occurs in puppies, especially in the larger breeds and where there is a shortage of calcium in the diet, when the ends of the long bones may separate from the central part.

The aim when treating a fracture is to position the broken parts in such a way that they set in the normal place (in correct alignment). They have to be immobilised to enable the setting to take place and to prevent pain.

The repair, which must be undertaken by a veterinary surgeon, can consist of external or internal fixation. The dog should receive professional attention immediately, if possible.

As an initial first aid measure, one should attempt to return the broken parts into position, and to retain them in place by bandages applied over cotton-wool-padded splints made of thin strips of wood or metal. If veterinary treatment has to be delayed, home treatment (i.e. first aid) is indicated. A dog with a fracture feels little pain if left undisturbed or if moved carefully.

There is no set time that broken bones take to recover, or for the dog to regain full use of the limb or damaged part of the body. The time involved depends on the type of fracture, on other injuries that may have also occurred and the age of the dog. On average a broken bone will be fully healed in 3 to 6 weeks, but the swelling

53

Frostbite

associated with bone healing may take considerably longer to disappear.

Greenstick fractures occur in young animals. The bones are bent rather than broken. Recovery, once treatment has been given, is usually fairly rapid (2 to 3 weeks).

Frostbite This is uncommon in dogs. If it does occur, it usually affects the ears and feet and must be treated quickly with warmth and massage. (Sudden heat should not be applied.)

The area should be wrapped in cotton wool after being dressed with acriflavine emulsion. The dog should be offered warm drinks. All parts of the body should be rubbed. Veterinary attention is essential if the part is not to be permanently damaged.

Fungal Eczema, *see* Ringworm.

Gallstones Generally believed not to occur in the dog.

Gangrene The death of some tissues of the body with degeneration of the tissues involved. This condition may be *primary*, where germs that cause the death of the tissues also cause the degeneration, or *secondary*, where germs cause degeneration in tissue killed by another cause, e.g. a burn.

Gangrene can also be divided into dry and moist forms. Dry gangrene occurs when the circulation is arrested and the part normally supplied dries and dies. Moist gangrene occurs when infection destroys an area and, as the name implies, the tissues soften and liquefy. In general, moist gangrene spreads, or tends to spread, while dry gangrene is restricted to a certain area.

Treatment consists of removal by surgical means of all dead tissue and the control of infection. This must be undertaken by a veterinary surgeon.

Gastric Ulcer Rarely seen in the dog.

Gastritis Inflammation of the stomach. A condition frequently seen in the dog, which shows symptoms of acute thirst, vomiting and often diarrhoea.

Treatment Keep the dog warm and quiet and give no food or cold water. Offer instead 5–20 ml (depending on the size of the dog) of warm water to which a small amount of sugar has been added—this should be offered once an hour. If the dog will drink this, but then vomits, the next dose should be offered in 2 hours' time. The liquid should be placed before the dog but it should not be forced to drink. If the dog will not drink it, the liquid should be removed until the time for the next dose.

Grass-Eating

There are two reasons why this condition can be dangerous: stomach damage and the risk of the infection spreading to other parts of the digestive tract, and reduction of the water and salt content of the dog's body after continuous vomiting.

Veterinary advice should be sought.

Gastro-Enteritis Inflammation of the stomach and intestines. The dog usually vomits, has diarrhoea and will not eat. Often the thirst is greatly increased. Treat as for gastritis (q.v.).

A veterinary surgeon should be consulted if recovery does not occur in 12 hours, or if the condition of the dog progressively worsens.

See also Haemorrhagic Gastro-Enteritis.

Gingivitis, *see* Gum.

Glandular Enlargement The dog has a large number of lymph nodes situated throughout the body. These have several functions, the most important probably being those of white blood cell formation and the 'filtering' of the fluid of the blood to remove infection and certain other unwanted matter.

When infection is present, these glands may swell. This can be used as a guide to determine if infection exists in a certain area of the body, as only those lymph nodes that are so working become increased in size.

Lymph nodes are often called glands. They can be felt at the angle of the neck and elsewhere in the body.

In generalised infection of the body, all lymphatic nodes are enlarged. In certain other diseases not connected with bacterial infection the glands may also increase in size.

See also Pseudo Hodgkin's Disease.

Glaucoma, *see* Eye.

Goitre Enlargement of the thyroid gland, which is situated low down in the neck. This condition, which is rare in the dog, is associated with an iodine deficiency. Veterinary advice is needed for a swelling in this site.

Grass-Eating This is common in dogs, and is usually due to the desire to fill the stomach so that it can then be emptied by vomiting. The most frequent causes are gastritis, digestive discomfort and worm infestation.

This is not a sign of abnormal appetite unless it occurs very often. However, it is sensible to ensure that the diet is balanced and that the dog is not suffering from internal parasites (q.v.).

Grass Seeds

Grass Seeds The seeds of certain grasses can cause trouble if they enter the tissues of the body. These seeds are usually long and pointed and become lodged in the ears, eyes, feet, coat and, more rarely, the penis or vulva.

Where these seeds become entangled in the hair of the coat they are usually easily detected and can be combed out without too much trouble. In other sites they may not be readily seen, and any sore in or near the ear, eye or foot should be cleaned and carefully examined to determine if it is caused by such a foreign body. Where a seed is present, it is usually possible to see one end as a small dark spike (the colour of the seed is darkened by the action of the liquid that accumulates round it) protruding from the sore.

When a seed enters the foot, it is possible for it to travel up the leg through the tissues, leaving a series or line of sores on the skin as it moves through the muscles or connective tissues.

Grass seeds in the penis or vulva are rarely visible, but the dog shows signs of great discomfort and constantly licks the part affected. Veterinary advice is essential.

If a seed is visible in any wound, it can usually be removed with tweezers after cleaning the part affected. Veterinary advice is always indicated.

Gripe, *see* Colic.

GUM

Bleeding, *see* Gingivitis.

Brown Mouth A condition where the gums become brown and have an unpleasant smell, associated with a general bacterial infection. Usually responds to antibiotic treatment.

Gingivitis Inflammation of the gums. In this condition, the gums become congested, red and 'angry-looking' along the margins and easily bleed when touched. The usual causes are scale formation on the teeth (q.v.), infection or a vitamin deficiency.

The teeth should be examined and scale removed if necessary. The mouth, especially the gums, should be washed in a salt solution or a weak solution of hydrogen peroxide (10 vol. hydrogen peroxide in an equal amount of water). The diet should be checked and adjusted if necessary to ensure that it is nourishing and provides a good and balanced supply of vitamins.

Growth on A hard, irregular-shaped growth is sometimes seen on the gum. An epulis is the most common form, and is usually seen in older dogs.

Haematoma

Where the growth is pedunculate (on a stalk), tie a piece of white cotton tightly round the stalk and leave it in place until the growth drops off. If this is not successful, surgery under anaesthesia may be needed. Veterinary advice should always be sought.

If such a growth has been removed, further growths may occur.

Other forms of growths may be found on the gums.

Gumboil A painful swelling of the gum caused by infection, usually from a decayed tooth. Such a tooth usually has to be removed, and antibiotics are necessary.

The mouth should be bathed in warm salt water. It may be necessary to lance an abscess (q.v.) that does not resolve.

Pyorrhoea Infection of the gums and tooth sockets with pus-producing organisms. If not treated, the teeth may become loose and eventually fall out. The infection starts around the teeth and spreads to the surrounding gums.

This condition usually occurs because scale or tartar forms on the teeth. If this is removed before infection sets in, the condition is unlikely to develop.

Treatment consists of teeth scaling to remove hard deposits, the removal of any teeth that are incapable of responding to treatment and the use of antibiotics to control infection.

If the dog's diet contains some hard matter that has to be chewed, this condition can be prevented.

Haematemesis The vomiting of blood. If the vomited blood is bright red, it indicates that this results from an injury to the stomach lining or oesophagus. However, if the blood is seen as small brown specks (like tealeaves) in the vomit, this is caused by inflammation of part or whole of the stomach lining membrane, where blood slowly seeps from the blood vessels into the stomach and there becomes partially digested.

Veterinary attention is essential. As a first aid measure give no food or liquid and keep the dog warm and quiet.

Haematoma A swelling caused by damage to a blood vessel, where blood collects at the point of damage but does not escape from the tissues. In the dog this occurs most commonly in the ear flap, where the swelling may reach a considerable size.

If small, a haematoma may resolve without treatment, but an ear may need surgical opening and the skin of that part may have

Haematuria

to be sutured back into position. The advice of a veterinary surgeon is required.

Take care that no further damage is done to the site, e.g. from self-inflicted injury by the dog.

Haematuria Blood in the urine. This may be due to a ruptured blood vessel, trauma, calculi, etc. (qq.v.).

Haemorrhage The following sections refer to the area from which the blood is seen to come.

BUCCAL Bleeding from the mouth, which can come from any part of the mouth or throat; usually from tooth sockets, inflamed or ulcerated gums, cut or ulcerated tongue or cheeks, or from cuts due to injuries. The latter are often caused by the dog chewing or playing with unsuitable sharp objects.

The cause must be determined. Where infection is found to be present, antibiotics are indicated. Small cuts and sores can be treated by syringing the mouth with a warm salt solution.

CEREBRAL, see Stroke.

EXTERNAL Bleeding from the surface of the body. In many cases this can be stopped by bandaging a pad of cotton wool into position over the area. If the bandage is tight, it is essential to ensure that the circulation in other parts of the body is not affected.

In other cases, where the bleeding is heavy, it can be controlled by applying direct pressure directly over the injured vessel or the spot where the blood is escaping. This can be done with the fingers or a tourniquet (q.v.). Where sizeable arteries are spurting blood, a tourniquet is essential. This should be slackened for a few seconds every 3 to 4 minutes if kept in place for any length of time. Heavy bleeding must have veterinary treatment as quickly as possible.

Once haemorrhage is controlled, after-treatment aims to overcome shock from loss of blood, and restore normal blood pressure.

INTERNAL Loss of blood into the body cavities. This usually follows an accident or injury.

It can be detected by signs of bodily weakness: the membranes of the eyes and mouth appear pale, the pulse is weak, and in some cases the dog sighs and moans.

Veterinary attention is essential.

NASAL This may result from injury, violent sneezing, growths, ulcers or worms in the nose. It can also occur where the blood pressure is raised and from certain infections.

Whenever possible, the cause should be determined. Where

blood is coming from one nostril only, this may be plugged with cotton wool held in place for some time by hand, or by means of a thin strip of adhesive plaster over the nostril. Ice placed over the nose will often help. It is necessary to ensure that where there is bleeding, this does not interrupt the dog's respiration. Fresh air is needed and the dog should be encouraged to relax with the neck extended. Excitement and exercise should be avoided while bleeding continues and, where possible, for a day afterwards.

TAIL   Injuries to the tip of the tail often cause bleeding that is difficult to control because the dog moves the tail and knocks it on various objects.

The cut should be cleaned, wrapped with gauze or clean white cloth, this covered with a thin layer of cotton wool and the whole enclosed in adhesive plaster. This dressing is designed to stop bleeding, but it must be light enough not to be too uncomfortable for the dog. The adhesive plaster keeps all in place and must be attached to the hairs above the dressing, thus preventing it from slipping off. Small pieces of plaster are of little use—a continuous roll is more efficient.

URINARY   Blood in the urine or a flow of pure blood, which can have many causes. All require veterinary treatment.

See also Haematemesis.

UTERINE   This should not be mistaken for the discharge that occurs when a bitch is in season.

The condition may be functional, where the hormonal control of the reproductive organs is disturbed but it can also follow injury, infection, tumours and after whelping (qq.v.).

In all cases, veterinary treatment is required.

Haemorrhagic Gastro-Enteritis   Inflammation of the stomach and intestines, where blood vessels are damaged and blood is seen in the motion. Vomiting, diarrhoea, listlessness and increased thirst are the common symptoms.

The dog should be kept warm, and all food and water temporarily taken away. A veterinary surgeon must be consulted.

Haemorrhoids (piles)   These do not occur in the dog. The condition often mistaken for haemorrhoids is that of *anal adenoma* (q.v.), a growth on the peri-anal region.

Hand-Rearing of Puppies   This is needed when a bitch is unable to feed her puppies for any reason, and is not difficult if common sense and care are used.

Hand-Rearing of Puppies

An alternative form of milk must be supplied. This may be cow's milk adjusted to suit the puppy, goat's milk, or special preparations made for this purpose and obtainable from chemists. If milk is used, a mixture of 0·125 litres of the milk plus one egg yolk is best.

It is essential to adopt a routine, so that the feeds are given regularly and the same type of milk is always used.

Every puppy is an individual. It is sensible to prepare more milk than is needed, and give as much as it will take in ten minutes, or until it falls asleep. The table is a guide to the amount of milk to prepare for each size of puppy per feed, together with the number of daily feeds.

Age of puppy	No. of 5 ml teaspoons for each feed				No. of feeds
	Toy	Miniature	Medium	Large	
birth–7 days	¼	½	1	1	10
8–14 days	½	1	2	2½	8
15–21 days	1	1½	2½	4	6
22–28 days	2	3	4	6½–8	5

For large puppies, one can sometimes use a baby's bottle with a small teat. Otherwise one must obtain a bottle made specifically for this purpose or get a plastic toy bottle made for dolls. These are usually made without an air inlet, so a small hole has to be made at the end. A plastic dropper can be used, but this tends to allow the puppy to swallow too much air. A glass dropper should not be used.

All spoons, bottles, teats, etc. must be thoroughly cleaned and sterilised before each feed.

The rearing of puppies in this way is not just a matter of supplying suitable milk. The milk must be given at blood-heat.

Puppies must be kept warm. The ideal is 90°–100°F (32°–37°C).

A puppy cannot empty its bladder or pass a motion when it is first born. This is stimulated by the licking of the mother. It is therefore necessary to stroke the stomach, hind legs and back of the hand-reared puppy before and after each meal. It should pass water each time, and a motion after every two or three meals.

The body should be wiped over after each meal with cotton

wool dipped in warm water to ensure that the coat is kept clean. The puppy must be dried before being returned to its bed.

As soon as a puppy can lap (at about $2\frac{1}{2}$ weeks of age), milk can be given in a shallow container. At 3 weeks of age solid food can be gradually added to the diet. Meat finely minced can be provided once a day at first (about $\frac{1}{2}$ teaspoonful), or a tin or jar of baby puree.

By 5 weeks, the puppy should be receiving 4 or 5 small meals a day—2 of these with a meat basis, the remainder being a milk mixture with some form of carbohydrate—cereal, biscuits, puppy meal, etc.

All changes in diet should be introduced gradually.

A hand-reared puppy may at times suck air into the stomach, which can cause pain. One or two drops of baby's gripe-water put on the puppy's tongue will usually bring it quick relief.

Hard-Pad Disease A disease (now infrequently seen) that is caused by a form of distemper virus. It is characterised by a high temperature in the early stages. Later the symptoms can be seen that give the name hyperkeratosis—the enlargement and hardening of the pads. The nose and eyelids may also be so affected. Dark patches are seen on the skin, especially of the ears and abdomen.

Clinically the disease cannot be distinguished from ordinary distemper until it has reached an advanced stage.

Treatment must be undertaken by a veterinary surgeon. Warmth, rest and quiet are essential (*see* Distemper).

Protection can be given by vaccines, etc. (*see* Immunity).

Hare Lip, *see* Hereditary Abnormalities.

Harvest Mites Small red mites, not usually visible with the naked eye, which are the larva of a species of *Trombidium*. They attack dogs, cats, humans and occasionally other animals.

In dogs the commonest site of attack is the feet, between the toes. Sores occur which later develop scabs. These are very irritant and make the dog lick and chew the foot.

Treatment consists of bathing the affected area with a parasiticidal solution and treating the sores with a soothing ointment.

Haw The nictitating membrane, or third eyelid.

HEART

Attack A sudden collapse (q.v.) due to heart and circulatory disturbance. The dog may have shown signs of coughing after exercise before the collapse.

Heat

Rest, freedom from external stimuli (noise, movement, changes of temperature, etc.) are essential. Veterinary advice must be obtained.

Where respiration is difficult, the tongue should be pulled as far as possible out of the mouth. The fumes of ammonia or smelling salts are useful if placed near the nose and mouth for a few seconds.

Disease The heart can be considered as a four-chambered pump, with valves between the chambers. Disease may affect any one of the chambers, the valves or the muscles that make the heart function, or the nerves that control the heart movement or beat.

For any heart disease, veterinary attention is essential. For first aid, the dog should be kept as quiet as possible, and stimuli of any type should be avoided.

Where the dog suffers from a continuous cough and veterinary advice is not immediately obtainable, a small amount (1–5 ml) of brandy may be given, depending on the size of the dog, and ¼–1 codeine tablet as an additional treatment while waiting for professional advice.

See also Pericarditis; Section 3.

Palpitation Unexpected increased action of the heart. The pulse, naturally, also has an increased rate. The dog is restless, pants, and may occasionally become unconscious.

See also Heart, Attack.

Heat, *see* Oestrus.

Heat-Stroke This condition, when occasionally seen in the dog, can result from its being over-exposed to sunlight (e.g. on a beach), or being left in a parked car without adequate ventilation.

Symptoms Vomiting or salivation, rapid pulse, weakness of the limbs, staggering gait and, finally, collapse (q.v.). The body temperature is raised, and skin normally white may become reddened.

Treatment Place the dog in cool and shade. Apply cold water, to which ice should be added if available, constantly to the head, neck and shoulders, by means of a cloth. When it has recovered, the dog should be dried, kept out of the sun and given plenty of cool water to drink.

Height This is the vertical distance from the ground to the highest point of the dog's withers, when the dog is standing with all four feet on level ground.

Hereditary Abnormalities

Hemiplegia Paralysis of one side of the body, including the limbs; rare in the dog.
See also Paralysis.
Hepatitis, Contagious Inflammation of the liver. This can have many causes. Veterinary advice is essential.
See Canine Virus Hepatitis; Leptospirosis.
Hereditary Abnormalities These are conditions that are not normal and arise from genetic origins. Many cause death before birth and are not easily identified.

Some abnormalities are encouraged by certain breed standards. Crooked fore-legs, excessively long ears, deep folds in the facial skin, large eyes, etc., all tend to enhance so-called 'beauty', but may produce trouble.

Very many conditions are recognised as being possibly caused by hereditary factors. Apart from those listed below, the following are also frequently encountered:

cryptorchidism (*see* Cryptorchid)
entropion (*see* Eyelid, Inverted)
hip dysplasia (q.v.)
hypoplasia of the reproductive organs
patella luxation (q.v.)
phimosis (*see* Penis)
scrotal and inguinal hernia (*see* Hernia)
umbilical hernia (may be hereditary or mechanical—*see* Hernia)

Dogs suffering from such conditions should not be used for breeding.

It is possible in some cases to determine if a dog or bitch is a carrier of an abnormal hereditary condition by test matings and the examination of the puppies so produced. In practice this is rarely carried out as the time and expense involved are extremely great. It is more common to attempt to 'breed out' such faults by testing all dogs that are to be used for breeding and using only those that are free from the condition.

CLEFT PALATE The two sides of the hard palate of the roof of the mouth are not properly united. This defect is most commonly seen in the short-nosed breeds. It is frequently associated with hare lip (q.v.). Affected puppies may pass milk from their nostrils when they suckle.

Hermaphrodite

Surgical correction is the only possible remedy, but it is not always successful.

HARE LIP   A defect, often hereditary, seen at birth, where the upper lips are not correctly joined at the mid-line. In some cases, it can be corrected surgically. It is usually not advisable to breed from dogs that show this condition.

PROGRESSIVE RETINAL ATROPHY   A form of night blindness, which the dog first shows by poor vision during the evening hours when the light is reduced. There may be an increase in the size of the pupil, but this is, in fact, a condition which takes several forms. The commonest has been outlined above while another type has no increase in the size of the pupil.

Retinal atrophy can also be caused by distemper or vitamin A deficiency, and may be associated with glaucoma.

UTERINE INERTIA   The inability to whelp at the expected time, because of lack of muscular contractions. This condition can also occur after injury, in old age, and when the bitch is unwell. Often a caesarean section is required to deliver the puppies.

Hermaphrodite   A dog that has some sexual organs of both sexes.

Hernia   The protrusion of an organ, or part of an organ, through the wall of the cavity in which the organ normally is contained. It is the term generally used for those conditions which involve the abdominal cavity.

The protruded organ, or part of an organ, is still enclosed in the membrane that lines the cavity in which the part is normally contained: i.e. the protruded part is enclosed in a sac of lining membrane when it enters the incorrect position. (In a rupture (q.v.), this lining membrane is torn.) *See* Figure 2.

The commonest forms (named after the site) are: diaphragmatic, inguinal, perineal and umbilical.

DIAPHRAGMATIC   Although this name is used, the condition is, strictly speaking, a rupture. It is seen in dogs that have suffered from a severe accident or fall. The diaphragm is torn and some of the abdominal contents enter the chest. Respiration is restricted, especially if the dog is held so that the hind-legs are higher than the fore-legs. Surgical repair is necessary.

INGUINAL   Seen most commonly in adult dogs of both sexes. A swelling occurs in the groin, usually at one side only. In the male, the hernia may involve the scrotum, in which case it is often termed a scrotal hernia. Surgical repair is needed.

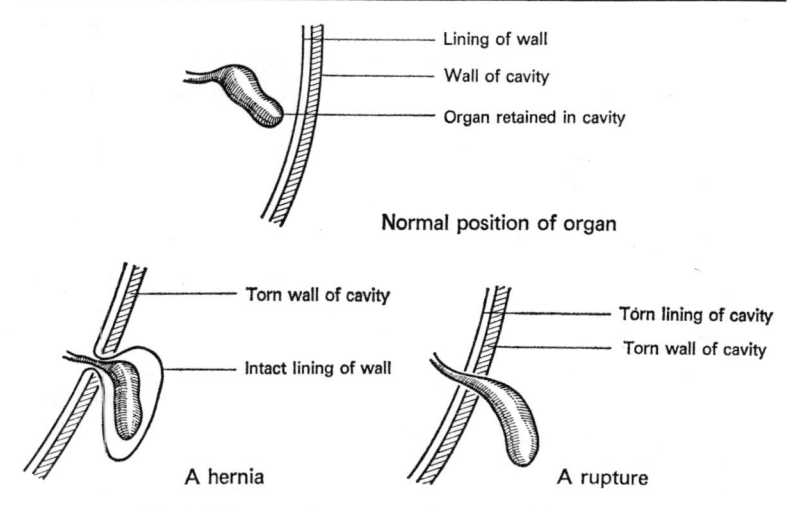

Figure 2 The difference between a hernia and a rupture

PERINEAL Seen mainly in elderly male dogs. A soft swelling occurs to one side of the anus. This condition is not as easy for a surgeon to repair as other types of hernia. Veterinary attention is essential.
UMBILICAL Usually seen in puppies, where the umbilical ring does not close or is damaged. A small bubble of fat forms at the site and can be felt; if pressed, it tends to enter the abdomen. When small, an umbilical hernia has little effect on the puppy. If large, it has to be corrected surgically.
Hiccough A spasm of the diaphragm, causing a sudden, jerky inspiration of breath, which is usually repeated at regular intervals. The condition is seen most commonly in puppies, where it is caused by a digestive disturbance.

In many cases, hiccoughs can be stopped by holding the dog so that he stands on the hind legs alone. Otherwise give a 5 ml dose of baby's gripe-water, or a pinch of bicarbonate of soda in a little milk.
Hidebound A term (not commonly used) which refers to conditions where there is a loss of subcutaneous fat and fluid so that the skin appears hard and is stretched over the dog's frame.
Hip Dysplasia The term used for a number of malformations of the hip joint. Some of these conditions are hereditary.

Hoarseness

The dog moves with a swaying gait, and may have difficulty in jumping. It is not usually noticed in a young puppy, but becomes apparent as the dog becomes heavier. It is commoner in the larger breeds.

The only way to confirm diagnosis is by X-ray, so that veterinary advice is essential.

Hoarseness   A husky and hollow bark, which is heard when the dog's throat is inflamed.

Hodgkin's Disease   A disease of humans, sometimes confused with pseudo Hodgkin's Disease of dogs.

Hookworm, *see* Parasites, Internal.

Hydrocele   An accumulation of fluid in the scrotum.

Hydrocephalus   A condition, seen mainly in the very young dog, where there is a collection of fluid in the membranes surrounding the brain. The head, especially the top of the skull, is large and rounded, and the puppy shakes it from side to side as though it were too heavy to hold up. The gait is unsteady, the puppy frequently walks in circles (generally in one direction), is constantly whining and crying, does not thrive and often has convulsions and dies.

There is no known treatment for this condition.

Hydrophobia   Fear of water. *See also* Rabies.

Hydrothorax   A collection of fluid within the pleural cavity. It is often one of the results of certain forms of pleurisy (q.v.).

Hyperkeratosis, *see* Hard-Pad Disease.

Hypodermic Syringe   An instrument used to give injections. It must be sterilised before use.

Hysteria   Excessive over-excitement from any cause. May be due to teething stress, shortage of calcium, toxaemia, nerve damage or mental instability. The condition should be treated as for fits (q.v.).

Icterus, *see* Jaundice.

Immunity   The term used to refer to the ability of the dog to resist certain specific infections, or the effects of certain poisons. It can be inherited, acquired naturally or induced artificially.

Inherited immunity is a resistance that is passed from dam to puppy. It may be an immunity that exists in all dogs, such as that which prevents dogs from becoming infected with tetanus, or it may be the resistance of an individual family or strain to a specific infection.

Immunity

Naturally acquired immunity occurs when a dog recovers from an infection and becomes able to resist any further attack by the same infective organism. This ability gradually weakens unless the animal concerned meets the infective organism at regular intervals.

Artificially acquired immunity can be either active or passive.

Active immunity is produced by injecting, or otherwise introducing into a dog, a vaccine or toxoid made specifically to produce resistance against a specific disease. As a general principle, these are made to combat diseases that are either widespread or a danger to human life. The commonly produced vaccines are against distemper, viral hepatitis, leptospirosis and rabies. In certain instances where a group of dogs suffer from an infection, it is possible to make an *autogenous vaccine*. This is a vaccine that is made from the germs that are isolated from the dogs concerned and protects them from the germ.

Actively immunised dogs are resistant to the disease against which they are protected for a long period, but this resistance gradually weakens unless the dog concerned meets the disease against which it is protected or is given additional doses of vaccine at regular intervals. Occasionally a dog is found that is incapable of reacting to a vaccine and therefore does not become immune when such a vaccine is used. It is possible that such dogs are naturally resistant to the disease concerned.

Passive immunity is a resistance to a specific disease, which is obtained by injecting a dog with serum from another dog that has been actively immunised against that disease. This serum (known as antiserum) is given in its natural form or as a concentrated extract. It contains antibodies which are the protective agent for that specific disease.

Unlike the resistance provided by active immunisation, passive immunity lasts only for a short while. Active immunity takes time to develop, while passive immunity is effective immediately after the injection is given.

Maternal, or colostral, antibodies are those that are passed from a dam to her puppies in her first milk (the colostrum). These provide the puppy with immunity against those diseases to which the dam has developed resistance. This maternal, or colostral, immunity is of short duration, usually 4–12 weeks.

See also Distemper; Leptospirosis; Vaccines; Viral Hepatitis.

Impetigo

Impetigo (a term not now commonly used)   This is a superficial infection of the skin, which is mainly seen in young dogs.

Bathing with a dog skin stimulant is usually sufficient to control the condition.

Impotence   Lack of virility. The term is commonly used to refer to the sexual ability of the male.

The condition may be due to mechanical impediment, functional impotence, failure due to over-use of stud dogs, etc., weakness following injury or ill-health, endocrine inactivity, castration, disease, atrophy, or non-descent of the testicles.

Where it is caused by over-use, rest from sexual activity is indicated. Otherwise, veterinary advice must be obtained. Good food, tonics, exercise and an interesting life all help to stimulate recovery.

Incontinence of Urine   The unexpected passing of water.

In puppies, this is usually due to nervousness, and wears off in time.

Causes   A variety of conditions, including cystitis, paralysis, bladder stones, tumours, enlarged prostate gland in the male.

Where this condition is caused by the bladder becoming over-full and the excess 'dribbling' out, it is essential to ensure that the bladder is emptied twice daily, using gentle pressure on the flanks, if this is possible.

Veterinary advice and treatment are essential.

Indigestion   The condition where the digestion of the food is disturbed. The term usually refers to disturbances associated with the stomach. Causes may be over-eating, ingestion of unsuitable food or food that is not correctly balanced. It may also occur where the digestive enzymes are not produced in the correct amount.

There may be associated vomiting, digestive discomfort, bad breath, poor health and loss of appetite.

In such a condition, it is essential to give the dog small meals frequently, to encourage exercise, to provide a varied diet, and to give a teaspoonful (5 ml) of gripe-water or sodium bicarbonate after each meal. *See also* Section 3.

If the dog suffers regularly from this condition it is essential to determine the cause and, whenever possible, remove or correct this.

Repeated attacks require veterinary attention.

Inflammation

Infertility   The inability to reproduce. This may be complete or partial.

Where a dog is completely infertile, the chance of a cure is uncertain. Where the reproductive powers are reduced, there is a fair chance of full recovery after treatment.

In all cases a detailed investigation into the cause is essential.

Male dogs which have been active and have fathered offspring but later cease to serve a bitch require good food, exercise and rest from sexual use.

Bitches that appear to be infertile may, in fact, be normal in all respects except that their reproductive cycle is different from other bitches in that the time of ovulation is very early or late. This means that mating at the usual time would be non-productive. A daily test of vaginal secretion during the season will soon demonstrate the time of ovulation and therefore the time of maximum receptivity.

See also Whelping.

Inflammation   The reaction of the body or part of the body to injury due to violence, infection, chemical agents, cold or heat. The blood vessels become enlarged and the tissues engorged with fluid and white blood cells. Bleeding may occur if blood vessels are damaged. Inflammation is characterised by pain, heat, swelling and redness. Loss of function often follows.

The results of inflammation are *resolution*, where the condition returns to normal; *suppuration*, where pus develops; *necrosis*, where the tissue concerned, or part of it, is destroyed; *gangrene* (q.v.), where all the tissue and that which surrounds the affected area dies; *ulceration*, where a shallow lesion develops on the surface of the area; or *granulation*, where the condition becomes chronic and there is an obvious thickening of the tissues.

Where inflammation occurs in a certain tissue it may be given a specific name: e.g. pneumonia = inflammation of the lungs, bronchitis = inflammation of the bronchi (qq.v.).

For home treatment it is essential to use common sense. If the dog is generally unwell it should be kept warm and quiet. Where a localised area is affected, this should be treated symptomatically—if moist, it should be dried with a wound dressing powder; if dry, it should be bathed with warm salt solution. If there is bleeding, this must be treated. Where the inflamed area is dirty, it must be cleaned. Where infection occurs, this must be combated.

Inguinal Hernia

In other words, the treatment depends on the symptoms, but it is essential that the area is protected from further infection and self-damage by the dog.
Inguinal Hernia, *see* Hernia.
Insect Stings, *see* Stings.
Interdigital Cysts, *see* Cysts.
Intussusception of the Bowel, *see* Bowel, Invagination of.
Invalid Food, *see* Section 3.
Irritation of the Skin The dog scratches, bites, licks, etc., although there appears to be no visible cause. The condition is seen mainly during hot weather or when the dog has been near a source of heat; it should not be confused with infestation by fleas, lice, allergic reactions, mange, etc.
See also Allergy; Eczema; Parasites, External.
Itch, *see* Eczema; External Parasites, External.
Jaundice The name given to the symptom of any disease in which the skin, the mucous membranes and the urine are yellow on account of the deposition of bile pigments in the tissues of the body. Can be 'obstructive' or 'non-obstructive'.

The *obstructive* form is caused by obstruction of the bile duct through inflammation, pressure due to growths, parasites, etc.

The *non-obstructive* form can be congestion of the liver, toxic agents in the blood, some forms of poisoning (e.g. phosphorus), etc.

Jaundice can be observed as the skin and mucous membranes turn yellow. The dog is listless, does not eat and is inclined to constipation; the urine tends to be concentrated and noticeably yellow.

Treatment must be undertaken by a veterinary surgeon, once the cause has been diagnosed. For first aid at home, it is essential to keep the dog warm, to restrict exercise, and to exclude fat from the diet.
Jaw, Overshot The lower jaw is too short for the upper jaw, so that the teeth of the lower jaw do not touch the inner surfaces of the upper incisors.
Jaw, Undershot A jaw where the lower incisors project beyond those of the upper jaw.
Kennels, Disinfection of All removable objects should be taken out of the kennels and scraped, cleaned and then treated with disinfectant. They should then be left out in an open place for as long as possible, as sunlight and fresh air are beneficial.

Knocked-Up Toe

The kennels themselves should be cleaned and washed, and air and light admitted. It is essential to use a disinfectant after everything movable has been taken out (including all dirt). The best is probably domestic bleach diluted as recommended, which can be applied to all surfaces.

Cement floors may be flooded with a solution of bleach or potassium permanganate, although the latter will tend to discolour the surface.

Chains, collars, leads, muzzles, and food and water containers should be washed and then soaked in disinfectant or bleach.

Waste matter should be burnt or placed in plastic sacks and then removed as quickly as possible.

Any traces of cleansing agent must be thoroughly washed away before the kennels are used again. The floors, walls and all equipment should be thoroughly rinsed with fresh water and then allowed to dry.

If a virus infection has been present in the kennels, all surfaces should be thoroughly washed in a 4 per cent solution of washing soda.

Kidney Disease   This is a common condition in the dog, and may be caused by infection or by damage to or an alteration in the tissues of the kidney.

The dog may have pain in the back, stiff hind legs or may pass large amounts of urine. However, other causes of the condition may lead to a restricted flow of urine.

As an aid to diagnosis, it is essential to take a urine sample for analysis in order to determine the correct treatment. The sample must be fresh.

Nephritis (inflammation of the kidneys) is common in urban dogs, and is often due to infection by *Leptospira* (*see* Leptospirosis).

Veterinary treatment is essential.

See also Uraemia; Section 3.

Kidney Stones (renal calculi), *see* Calculus.

Knocked-Up Toe   This condition is most commonly seen in racing Greyhounds. The toe affected is misplaced and swollen, and the joint nearest the end of the foot is dislocated. Pain is usually shown. Thickening and fibrous tissue may later develop.

Treatment is usually to amputate the digit. This has no lasting ill-effect on the dog, does not interfere with movement, and allows it to run and act normally.

Knuckling Over

Splinting, internal fixation of the joint and massage can also be used, but may not be successful in repairing the damage.

Knuckling Over A term used to describe a condition where the carpus, or wrist joint, is abnormal and allows the joint to fall forward when the dog is standing. Veterinary attention is needed, and the condition often has to be corrected surgically.

Labial Eczema A condition seen in these dogs which have a marked labial crease (or fold) at the side of the lower jaw, e.g. Spaniels.

The fold tends to collect dirt and become moist; the ensuing warmth encourages the development of infection. The result is inflammation and a strong, unpleasant smell.

The fold should be cleaned, the hair clipped away, washed with 10 vol. hydrogen peroxide, dried and then powdered with a wound dressing powder or bicarbonate of soda powder. This treatment should be repeated twice daily for 5 days. If the condition does not improve quickly, veterinary advice must be obtained.

Labour, *see* Whelping.

Lactation The secretion of milk, or the period during which a bitch produces milk. It starts soon after whelping, and continues in the normal bitch until the demand by the puppies ceases.

DEFECTIVE This can be due to infection, inflammation, injury, poor nutrition or the inability of the dam to supply enough milk for the number of puppies she is nursing.

The bitch often appears healthy, but the puppies are not able to receive sufficient milk. They seem weak, listless, and utter a piercing and plaintive cry. Often the dam rejects one or more puppies (she does not allow them to feed).

The cause of the condition must be determined. The puppies should be helped by supplying additional food (*see* Hand-Rearing of Puppies).

Liberal food, supplied frequently in small amounts, and milk should be given to the bitch. Food supplements of any form are useful. She should be encouraged to drink as much as possible.

EXCESSIVE The dam produces more milk than the puppies require; the milk glands become distended and inflamed and, if not treated, possibly infected.

The bitch is restless, and the mammary glands are swollen and hard to the touch. The puppies often appear to be unhappy, and cry continuously, as they are unable to suckle normally.

If the milk supply is quite abnormally excessive, some of the milk should be removed by stroking the milk glands. The bitch should be given less water, the usual amount of food, and increased exercise. A small amount of Epsom salts added to the food or water also helps.

Lameness The inability to move in a normal manner. The term usually refers to conditions of the limbs or back.

CAUSES The number is almost unlimited: the commonest are cuts, bites, grazes, fractures, dislocation of joints, rheumatism, arthritis, bone abnormalities, slipped disc, thorns or foreign bodies in the foot, and interdigital cysts.

It is sometimes difficult to determine which leg is lame when the condition is slight. It is helpful to know that a lame dog tends to nod its head downward when walking. This dropping of the head occurs when the sound leg is put to the ground in fore-leg lameness, and when the lame leg is put to the ground in hind-leg lameness.

Treatment must depend on the cause. Where the surface of the skin is involved, it is important to stop the dog licking a sore or wound. Surface lesions should be bathed with warm water to which salt has been added—the amount is not important, it is the drawing action of the salt in the water that is helpful.

Laryngitis Inflammation of the larynx, which can occur at any time, but is most commonly seen in spring and autumn. The condition usually causes a harsh dry cough, while the dog appears quieter than usual and eats less.

Warmth, limited exercise and soft food all alleviate the condition, while a mixture of equal quantities of raw white of egg, water and sugar given in small amounts at frequent intervals helps where the cough is very pronounced.

Veterinary treatment must be obtained if the cough remains for more than 2 days or where several dogs are affected.

This condition is often seen in dogs that have been boarded out at a kennel.

Lead Poisoning, *see* Poisoning.

Length of Life, *see* Age.

Leptospirosis This disease is caused by species of *Leptospira*. The principal ones are *L. canicola* and *L. icterohaemorrhagiae*.

L. canicola causes a disease of the kidneys which can occasionally lead to almost immediate death. However, it normally produces a

Leucorrhoea

chronic kidney weakness which may shorten the dog's life. The disease is spread through the urine, and is common in towns. It can be transmitted to human beings causing a mild illness, canicola fever.

L. icterohaemorrhagiae causes a serious and often fatal illness which usually affects the liver and kidneys. Jaundice is often seen. The disease is more common in country districts. Infection is spread by rats and direct contact and can cause a serious disease in man—Weil's disease.

These diseases must be treated by a veterinary surgeon.

It is possible and sensible to immunise dogs against leptospirosis; annual boosters are required to maintain protection (*see* Vaccines).

Leucorrhoea A pale grey, yellow or white discharge from the vulva, which occurs with inflammation of the uterus (q.v.).

Lice Small brown or blue-grey parasites which attack the skin of the dog. They move slowly and, although they are found throughout the coat, it is easier to recognise any infestation if the edges of the ear flap are carefully examined with a hand lens. Their eggs (called nits) are stuck to the hairs.

Two species occur on the dog: *Ligognathus piliferus* and *Trichodectes canis*. The latter is the intermediate host (carrier) of the tapeworm *Dipylidium caninum* (*see* Parasites, Internal).

Treatment consists of baths, powders or sprays, all intended to spread a drug throughout the coat and over the skin. This has to be repeated at intervals of about 5 days for 3 or 4 weeks to ensure that all eggs are killed as they hatch.

Licking, Scratching and Rubbing, prevention of. Increase exercise in order to distract the dog.

Keep the dog cool, as heat increases the irritation of sores and injuries.

Bandage the site so that the dog cannot touch it.

Make an Elizabethan collar. This is a circle of cardboard or leather which is cut so that when it is attached to the collar it projects forward between the dog's mouth and the affected site. Probably the easiest to make and the most efficient is made from a child's plastic bucket. Cut the bottom out and insert the dog's head into the opening. The bucket projects forward and is then attached to the collar.

Lightning Stroke The possibility of a dog being struck by lightning is remote. Should it happen, treat as for burns (q.v.).

Lungs

Liniment This is a preparation that is applied externally with friction for the treatment of sprains and bruises and other inflammatory processes.
LIPS
Cracked The cracks are usually seen along the edges of the lips, which become dry and thick, so that further cracks develop.
The affected parts should be gently cleaned with warm water to soften scabs, etc. Where hair is covered or surrounded by exudate, this should be clipped away to prevent recurrence. The areas should be covered with a soothing cream.
Sore Sores or ulceration of the lips may be caused by ill-health of other parts of the body, infection of the gums or teeth, injury, or a vitamin deficiency.
The cause should be discovered and treated. Give vitamin supplements to the dog's diet, and bathe the area affected with a weak solution of hydrogen peroxide (equal quantities of 10 vol. hydrogen peroxide and water).
See also Labial Eczema.

Liver, Inflammation of (Hepatitis) This condition may be caused by an infectious disease, poisoning (e.g. Phosphorus, q.v.), circulatory disturbance, etc.
Vomiting may occur; jaundice often becomes apparent; pain may be felt in the region of the liver.
Treatment depends on the cause, and should be undertaken by a veterinary surgeon. The diet should be controlled to ensure that the fat content is reduced or eliminated.
See also Canine Virus Hepatitis; Leptospirosis.
Lockjaw, *see* Tetanus.
Loss of Appetite, *see* Appetite, Decreased.
Loss of Balance, *see* Ataxia.
Loss of Hair, *see* Alopecia; Eczema; Parasites, External; Ringworm.
LUNGS
Congestion of The presence of an increased amount of blood in one or both lungs. This condition may be caused by infection, over-exertion, chemical irritants, smoke, or the passage of liquid into the lung instead of the digestive tract.
The condition is one that often develops into pneumonia. Veterinary attention is essential.

75

Luxation

Symptoms Rapid, distressed breathing, often with the head held extended and the mouth partly open. In some cases the dog sits with the fore-legs held wide apart. The eyes are often bloodshot, the pulse weak, and the temperature may be raised.
Home treatment Enforced rest in a warm but well-ventilated room is essential. 5 ml of brandy may be given in a little water or milk.
A veterinary surgeon must be called as quickly as possible.
Inflammation of, *see* Pneumonia.

Luxation, *see* Dislocations.
Maggots, *see* Fly Attacks.
Mammary Tumours, *see* Tumours.
Mammitis Inflammation of the mammary glands (*see* Mastitis).
Mange A contagious, parasitic skin disease occurring in several forms, each caused by a particular type of mite. The most common are *sarcoptic* and *otodectic*.

The mites bite into the skin and feed on blood and newly formed tissue. They are round or oval in shape, have spines and bristles and are too small to be seen easily. Eggs hatch in 3 to 7 days. The entire life-cycle can be as short as 7 days.

The dog suffering from such an attack has an irritant skin and loss of hair, with dry scurfy flakes in the part of the coat that remains. The skin often appears red when the dog has been near a source of heat. The areas attacked depend on the type of mite.

Treatments using baths, powders or sprays are effective against all forms of mange except demodectic. All treatment must be repeated twice weekly for several weeks. Drugs in tablet form are also effective but in some dogs they have undesirable side-effects.

When treating these infestations, ensure that the bathing, powdering, or whatever method is used, is carried out very thoroughly. If such treatment is not applied efficiently, treatment will only prolong the attack.

Mange mites cannot survive for long periods without a dog, but bedding, runs, pens or exercise yards must be thoroughly cleaned daily during the period of treatment.

Veterinary advice is essential.

If a dog is suffering from any form of mange, the owner must insist that the type of mange be determined. Should the owner suffer from any kind of rash or irritation, the family doctor should be consulted immediately.

Mating

The following is a brief alphabetical outline of some of the commoner types of mange and mange mites that attack dogs.

CHEYLETIELLA (various species) These can infest dogs, usually with no visible effect, but they cause a very irritant rash in humans. In humans, this is self-limiting unless the carrier (in this case, the dog) is constantly present. The owner therefore suffers from the infection on the dog.

DEMODECTIC This differs from other types of mange in that it is not readily spread from one dog to another. Close bodily contact is needed, and it is thought that a predisposition or other related factor is associated with the spread. Treatment is not always successful, while in the 'cured' animal it is possible that the parasite is still present but inactive. It is sometimes called follicular mange.

OTODECTIC This infects dogs' ears, producing irritation, the secretion of wax, earache, etc.

PSOROPTIC This affect rabbits, but has been known to attack the skin on the face of dogs.

SARCOPTIC (can also affect man) The sites on the dog most commonly infested are the ear edges, the axilla (arm pit) and the abdomen, although the entire body may be involved.

Marie's Disease In this condition, new bone is deposited on existing bones. Tumours, hormonal imbalance, vascular changes, and roundworm infestation have all been suggested as possible causes.

Mastitis Inflammation of the mammary (milk) glands. This condition is seen mainly in the bitch when she is producing, or about to produce, milk. The glands become hot, reddened, hard and sore. If milk is being produced, this may cease or be curtailed. Naturally the bitch appears distressed.

One or more glands may be involved. Puppies feeding from a bitch so affected usually do not thrive, may cry continuously, and lose weight. Hand-rearing may have to be started (*see* Hand-Rearing of Puppies).

The bitch requires veterinary treatment. The puppies should not be allowed to feed while she is ill. However, if she becomes distended with milk, this should be drawn away by stroking with the hand or by using a breast pump.

Mating The act of sexual intercourse. In an 'arranged' mating it is usual, and better, to take the bitch to the dog.

Meningitis, Cerebral

The bitch will receive the dog only during the 10th–12th day of oestrus (season). She must be healthy, not tired, and rested before mating. Sometimes it is arranged for her to be mated twice, at an interval of 1 or 2 days, to try to ensure conception.

During mating, the two dogs become 'tied' (*see* Tie) and cannot separate for a period.

See also Sterility.

Meningitis, Cerebral Inflammation of the meninges of the brain. This condition is usually caused by infection, the after-effects of infection or by injury.

For those giving home treatment, the advice for fits (q.v.) may be followed. The advice of a veterinary surgeon is essential.

Metritis, *see* Uterus, Inflammation of.

Milk The milk of the bitch is stronger and richer than that of the cow, as the following table shows:

	Cow's	Bitch's
water	87·4%	66·3%
fats	4·0	14·8
soluble salts and sugar	5·0	2·9
casein and insoluble salts	3·6	16·0

The milk of the goat is very similar to that of the bitch.

See also Hand-Rearing of Puppies.

DEFECTIVE SECRETION, *see* Lactation, Defective.

EXCESSIVE SECRETION, *see* Lactation, Excessive.

MILK FEVER, *see* Eclampsia.

Misalliance The mating of a bitch when this is not planned or wanted by the owner.

Unwanted pregnancy in the dog can be stopped by an injection given by a veterinary surgeon, provided that this injection is given within 36 hours of the mating.

There are, however, possible side effects following such an injection, as the season itself is usually prolonged, there is a risk of disturbance of the hormonal control of reproduction (especially if the injection has to be given more than once to any bitch) and certain skin conditions can be aggravated.

In general it is a lesser risk to have the injection than to allow the bitch to have puppies, but it is unwise to rely on injection instead of controlling the bitch while she is in season.

Miscarriage The premature ending of pregnancy because of

injury, infection, hormonal imbalance, etc., where the immature puppy is expelled from the bitch.
This is relatively rare in the dog. Veterinary advice is essential.
See also Abortion.

Molar Abscess Another name for dental fistula (q.v.).

Monorchid A male dog which has only one testicle. This name is also used (although not stricly correctly) for a dog with only one testicle in the scrotum, the other being retained in the abdomen.

In certain cases this condition may be inherited.

Moulting Most dogs shed their hair twice a year, in the autumn and spring. This moulting appears to be controlled by the length of day. It is for this reason that some dogs which live in surroundings where there is warmth and many hours daily of artificial light tend to have irregular, or continuous moults.

The period of coat-shed is usually about 14 days.
See also Alopecia.

Mouth, *see* Gums; Lips.

Muscle Wasting This can occur in any part of the body where muscles are not used or are unable to function. The condition is seen in a dog that has been ill for a long period and so has not been exercised, or where a limb or other part of the body has been splinted or made immobile for any reason. In this type of case the muscles gradually return to normal function and shape as exercise is increased and the part used.

In cases where wasting occurs due to lack of use because the nerve or blood supply is restricted or damaged, recovery is slow. Where such supply is severed, it is often impossible to obtain a response to treatment.

Veterinary advice should always be obtained. Massage, alternate hot and cold compresses, good food and encouragement to use the part affected all aid recovery.

Muzzling a Dog Special muzzles may be obtained for dogs. If it is necessary to muzzle a dog, perhaps because it has been injured, and it is too frightened to be easily handled, and such a muzzle is not available, a good temporary one can be made from a length of wide bandage, a football bootlace or other soft but strong material. The length should be about 1·5 m (5 ft). Hold one end of this in the left hand, together with the dog's collar. With the right hand, grasp the middle of the tape and, pulling the tape to the

Nails

left of the dog's neck, wind it twice round the dog's muzzle, taking care not to get bitten. Pull the loose end of the tape to the right side of the dog's neck and tie it to the end being held in the left hand in such a way that the tape is behind the ears and tight enough to prevent the part round the mouth from slipping. When correctly applied, this muzzle prevents the dog from opening its mouth, but does not cause it any harm. Once it is in place, take care to ensure that the dog does not remove the tape with its front feet.

NAILS

Cutting This cannot be undertaken safely with scissors; nail-cutters should be used. Where the nails are white, the procedure is simple as the quick can be seen and the nail may be cut to within $\frac{1}{16}$ inch (2 mm) from it; but if the nail is darker coloured or black, the quick is not so easily visible and the first nail must be cautiously cut, a little at a time. The dog will wince when the cutters are getting near the sensitive part. Once one is cut, it is less difficult to cut the rest, as they may be shortened in the same proportion as the first.

See also Dew-Claws.

Injuries to These may be caused by defective action of the foot, or by injury.

Dogs who limp or have some other defective action tend to wear away their nails unevenly. Where this occurs to such an extent that one or more nails are excessively shortened, the quick may be damaged. It is also possible that other nails may not be worn away at all and so become over-long. These are often curved and eventually re-enter the foot and cause sores.

Where nails are the normal length, one or more may be damaged, usually by becoming trapped in a crack during exercise. The nail is either broken, or is torn away from the nail-bed.

Treatment consists of cutting nails that are too long, removing torn pieces of nail where such damage exists, and providing exercise on soft ground where the nail is too short. If there are sores, these should be bathed in warm water into which a small amount of Epsom salts has been added (about a teaspoonful in 0·5 litre of water). It is easiest if the dog is made to stand with the affected foot in a bowl into which the liquid is poured. The foot should be soaked for about 5 minutes two or three times a day. If at all possible the foot should not be bandaged, although the dog must be prevented from licking the sores.

Nervousness

Where injury is bad or recovery is slow, a veterinary surgeon should be consulted.

Where infection is present, an antibiotic should be used.

If the dew-claw is broken, this usually occurs through the quick (the part where the blood-vessels, nerves and soft tissue are situated). The broken piece must be cut away at the point of breakage with one rapid cut with nail-cutters. Any haemorrhage should be controlled by applying dry cotton wool and a bandage.

Nasal Discharge   A discharge from the nostrils is usually caused by infection, either directly attacking the nasal region or entering this region because of foreign bodies (e.g. grass seeds), cold, dust or chemicals, or through an illness affecting the body generally.

Note that a dog with a discharge from the nostril which is clear, slight and watery in appearance may be in perfect health.

The dog with a nasal discharge usually sneezes; the discharge is yellow, white or green, and a swelling of the throat glands can be felt at each side of the jaw below the ear.

The dog should be kept away from cold or draughts, exercise should continue but should not be excessive, and inhalants should be used. Friar's Balsam, Vick, or any human nasal spray may be used.

Any general infection should be treated.

If there is distemper, treat as for that disease (q.v.).

Nasal Polypus   A growth, usually with a narrow neck, which forms in the nasal passage causing irritation, sneezing, snorting and a purulent discharge which may be tinged with blood.

Treatment consists of the surgical removal of the growth, which is often carried out by ligating its stalk. Naturally, veterinary attention is essential.

Necrosis   The death of tissue on a scale that is visible to the naked eye.

Nephritis   Inflammation of the kidneys (*see* Kidney Disease).

Nervousness   Causes may be bad management, improper training, poor health, bad sight or hearing, or poor diet. It can occasionally be of genetic origin.

Treatment depends on the cause. Where possible, this should be corrected. In every case, careful handling and training assists. If the dog and the owner can attend a school for dog training, this is ideal.

See also Section 2, 'Canine Behaviour Patterns'.

Nettle-Rash

Nettle-Rash, *see* Allergy; Stings.

Neuralgia The literal meaning is 'nerve pain' and the term is applied to pain for which no cause can be discovered. The name is now rarely used, as the cause of pain can usually be diagnosed.

Rest and warmth are essential for treatment. Soluble aspirin may be given, 100–300 mg every 4 hours depending on the size of dog.

Neuritis Inflammation affecting the nerves. It may be followed by paralysis or lack of sensation of the part of the body served by the nerve.

Nipples, Sore, *see* Teats, Sore.

Nose, Cold A normal healthy dog has a cold, moist nose. This may become dry and warm under stress, ill-health or excessive exercise.

Nose, Hot and Dry This may be a sign of ill-health, but it can also frequently occur in the healthy dog. Usually it is associated with stress; thus a dog that wants to empty its bladder but is unable to go outside may have a dry, hot nose.

Nose-Bleeding, *see* Haemorrhage, Nasal.

Nursing If a dog is not well, the following points should be noted.

A dog requires a dry, draught-proof place for rest with light and a fairly constant temperature (*see* Section 2, 'The Requirements of the Dog').

The dog itself and the kennel or living area must be kept clean at all times.

A dog requires pleasant surroundings.

All things used for the dog or for its treatment must be thoroughly clean. Even the owner's hands should be washed before and after handling the dog when it is ill.

The patient must be allowed to rest. It should be left undisturbed except for feeding, treatment and cleaning. Children may be allowed to 'visit' their dog only at prescribed intervals.

Treatment must be carried out thoroughly, regularly, and at the correct time.

Fresh clean water must always be available, unless your veterinary surgeon advises otherwise.

Dressings, bandages, etc. should not be reused unless boiled. Dressings that have been soiled by a wound or discharge must never be reused.

The advice of the veterinary surgeon must be followed com-

Oedema

pletely, even if this means getting up in the middle of the night. *See also* Whelping.

Nymphomania Excessive sexual desire in the bitch. The condition usually leads to frustration and therefore bad temper.

The cause is an imbalance of sexual hormones and is often related to dysfunction of the ovary.

Veterinary attention is essential. Sedatives and hormones can be used, but in many cases surgical removal of one or both ovaries or the spaying of the bitch is necessary.

Obesity (Overweight) This condition is usually due to overeating, under-exercise, improper diet or disease (e.g. diabetes mellitus, q.v.). There may, in a few cases, be a hereditary link.

The normal dog of normal weight should have a thin layer of fat under the skin which can be used as a guide—the ribs of a dog that is not overweight can be felt easily when it is stroked.

To slim an overweight dog it is first essential to ensure that the cause is not due to ill-health—any illness must be treated.

Provided the dog is not sick, the amount of food eaten should be gradually reduced and the diet gradually changed so that it contains less carbohydrate (*see* Section 3, 'Feeding a Dog').

The emphasis on the word 'gradual' is deliberate. The diet is improved but reduced in amount. At the same time, exercise should be gradually increased.

Loss of weight may not start immediately such measures are commenced. However, over a period of several weeks, the change will be noticeable. It is sensible to weigh the dog every second week to check the amount lost (*see* Weighing a Dog).

Special diets made for overweight dogs are available in the form of tinned food.

Oedema Puffiness, or diffused swellings about the body or legs, caused by a collection of fluid in the connective tissue under the skin, the abdominal cavity, chest cavity or any organ. This fluid comes from the blood or lymph vessels.

The cause may be severe bruising, damage to blood vessels, circulatory disturbances due to imbalances of the salt content of the blood, heart disease, failure of certain organs to function properly, the arrest of local circulation—e.g. when a leg is bandaged too tightly without the foot being covered, so that the foot tends to swell—and, in the lungs, after the animal has been exposed to smoke or intense dust.

Oedema of the subcutaneous connective tissue causes swelling under the skin which 'pits' on pressure; when the pressure is removed, the depression refills only slowly.

Treatment must depend on the cause. However, massage and movement of the limbs, if these are affected, help. Too tight bandages should be eased at once. Where respiration is affected, fresh air assists.

Oestrus (also known as heat or season) The period of sexual activity in the bitch, which usually occurs twice a year, during which time she will accept the male.

Just before each oestrus, her vulva becomes swollen and there is a bloodstained discharge. At this stage the male is attracted, but the bitch does not allow him to mate. About a week later the discharge loses most of its blood content and becomes yellowish. The male is then encouraged to mate. This stage lasts approximately a week, after which the vulva gradually returns to a normal size and the discharge ceases by the end of a further 7 days.

A bitch normally has her first oestrous period at about 6 months, but this can vary considerably.

See also Mating; Sterility.

Ophthalmia Inflammation of all the structures of the eye (q.v.).

Orchitis Inflammation of the testicles. This may result from injury, infection or, occasionally in old age, from constitutional causes.

The testicles become swollen and very painful, the scrotum is red and shiny. The dog walks and sits with difficulty.

Rest is essential. Soluble aspirin (100–600 mg) given three times a day, according to the size of the dog will help until veterinary advice can be obtained.

Orphaned Puppies, *see* Hand-Rearing of Puppies.

Osteomalacia A disease of the adult which is analogous to rickets in the immature animal. The bones become soft and brittle and there is pain and weakness, while the dog may show signs of exhaustion. The disease has been called 'rubber jaw' as there is a tendency for the lower jaw to be most commonly affected.

Veterinary advice must be obtained.

Osteosarcoma A malignant bone tumour (*see* Tumours, malignant).

Otitis (inflammation of the ear), *see* Ear, Canker.

Paralysis

Otorrhoea (inflammation of the ear), *see* Ear, Canker.
Ovarian Cysts   The term used for cysts that develop in the ovary. The condition often causes nymphomania (q.v.).
Overshot Jaw, *see* Jaw.
Palpitation, *see* Heart.
Pancreas   A gland lying in the abdomen that produces digestive juices which are liberated into the small intestine. These aid digestion. In addition, this gland produces hormones which affect the control of the body fluids and their composition. This is particularly significant as this gland controls the balance of body 'sugar' through the production of insulin.
See also Diabetes Mellitus; Pseudo-Diabetes.
Paralysis   The term used where a nerve controlling a muscle, or group of muscles, does not work; or where, because of nerve damage, there is a loss of sensation.

Where paralysis affects one side of the body only, it is termed *hemiplegia*; *diplegia* refers to both sides. In *paraplegia*, all parts of the body behind a certain point in the back are paralysed—this usually includes the functioning of the bladder and rectum.

Paraplegia is probably the most usual form of paralysis in the dog. Long-backed breeds are the most commonly affected. The site is usually the lumbar region of the spinal cord, and the paralysis is caused by an injury or a 'slipped disc'.

Localised paralysis also occurs where injury to a nerve affects the function or sensation of a limb or area. *Radial paralysis* is the most commonly seen form of this type of malfunction. Here, injury to the radical nerve in the fore-leg prevents the moving forward (extension) of the lower part of the leg. The elbow joint is held lower and the toes tend to rest on the ground pointing backwards. Recovery from this type of injury is possible, although the process is slow.

Veterinary treatment is essential. The basic rules of nursing (q.v.) apply.

Instruction in methods of emptying the bladder of a paraplegic dog should be obtained from the veterinary surgeon, and this emptying carried out twice daily. The emptying of the rectum is not so important—provided a motion is passed once or twice a week, there need be no worry.

The dog should be confined to an area just large enough to lie fully extended. If it cannot move at all, it should be turned over

Paraphimosis

so that it lies on alternate sides every 6 hours to aid circulation and to prevent the development of bed sores.

Foam rubber pads or double nylon fur fabric make a good bed as they are soft and can be easily cleaned. But care must be taken to ensure that they are not chewed or eaten.

Food should be supplied in small quantities, as the lack of exercise reduces the amount required. If the dog is given too much it increases in weight, and this delays recovery.

Spend time twice or thrice daily in helping the dog. The limbs should be massaged, and the abdomen supported for short periods so that the limbs can swing and thus help to maintain circulation and muscle strength. Infra-red irradiation of the spine may help. Warm or hot baths may occasionally be recommended.

Recovery from such injuries is not certain and, where it does occur, is slow. As a rough guide, a dog should be treated for 3 weeks before deciding that recovery is unlikely. Usually by this time any signs of improvement are obvious, and therefore the treatment must be continued.

Paraphimosis, *see* Penis.

Parasites, External   These live on, or in, the surface area of the skin. To remove these parasites, treat the dog at intervals to ensure that the parasite life-cycle is completely destroyed, otherwise the condition may recommence.

Baths, powders that are dusted onto the body, sprays, shampoos and tablets can all be used to treat dogs with these parasites but care must be taken to ensure that the directions are correctly followed.

See Fleas; Harvest Mites; Lice; Mange; Ringworm; Ticks.

Parasites, Internal   These live within the body. The following are some of the most common internal parasites that infest the dog.

COCCIDIA   A microscopic protozoal parasite which affects the small intestine, causing coccidiosis.

Although this condition occurs more often in warmer climates, it appears to be becoming more common, especially in dogs kept in 'closed communities' such as breeding kennels. A lack of hygiene leads to the development and spread of the disease.

Usually young puppies are affected—the symptoms include bloody diarrhoea, loss of appetite and loss of weight. Occasionally they may die. The infestation is less serious in adult dogs, but they may become carriers and so spread the disease.

Parasites, Internal

Correct diagnosis, with an examination of the faeces under a microscope, and accurate treatment are essential. Great care must be taken to ensure that the kennels and all equipment are kept clean. A high standard of hygiene is necessary if the disease is to be controlled.

HOOKWORMS The type seen in Britain are usually not serious (and relatively rare), but the form which occurs in other countries may cause anaemia.

WHIPWORMS These are seen in England and may become more common.

Hookworms and whipworms are not usually visible to the naked eye. Treatment is by tablets given at intervals of 2 or 3 weeks.

ROUNDWORMS (Ascarids) The adult worm lives in the intestines. If present in large numbers, they can cause severe ill-health or, in young puppies, an intestinal obstruction. The larval stages migrate through the tissues, especially the lungs, liver, brain or eye. Damage can be caused by this migration. In the pregnant bitch, the larvae of certain types migrate into the developing puppies and these show signs of infestation at 3–5 weeks of age.

The larvae of *Toxocara* can attack humans, but only babies up to a few months old. It is therefore sensible to worm all dogs, especially young ones, when there is a small baby in the house.

Treatment for roundworms is usually in the form of tablets or medicine which is given at 6, 9, and 12 weeks of age, at 5 months and then yearly, although not every owner takes this amount of care.

TAPEWORMS The segments of these worms are often seen in the motions, if infestation is present. These segments may be attached to the hairs around the anus—they may become dry and look like grains of rice. All canine tapeworms have a life-cycle which includes a host other than the dog. Treatment must therefore be directed against the worm and the intermediate host.

The commonest tapeworm is *Dipylidium caninum*, whose intermediate host is the flea and the louse. Treatment for infestation is therefore against the worm and the ectoparasites. Other tapeworms have their intermediate stage in rats, mice, rabbits, hares and sheep.

Treatment is not always easy. Unless the drug used destroys the worm completely, it is essential to check the motions after treatment to ensure that the entire worm is eliminated. The head is the

Parturient Eclampsia

smallest part, and is easily overlooked when examining the remains of an excreted worm—it looks like a small round blob at the end of a narrower neck.

Parturient Eclampsia, *see* Eclampsia.

Patella Luxation (also known as slipped patella, or kneecap) In this dislocation of the kneecap, it moves towards the body midline and so interrupts the proper movement of the knee joint. If dislocated, the patella may reposition itself or it may be replaced by a person by extending (pulling) the leg. However, once displaced, there is often a weakness which allows the condition to recur.

Where the condition is severe, the function of the leg may be completely interrupted. In many cases, surgery is the only method of permanent correction.

The cause is usually the poor development of the groove in the end of the femur (the long bone from the hip to the knee), or of the ridges alongside this groove.

The condition is rarely seen in very small puppies. It is only after growth has occurred and increased weight is placed on the knee joint that symptoms develop.

The tendency towards patella luxation is often inherited. Affected dogs should not be used for breeding.

Pediculi (Lice) These cause a contagious, parasitic disease also known as 'pediculosis' (*see* Lice).

PENIS

Balanitis An inflammation of the mucous membrane of the glans penis or the whole of the penis, usually causing coloured (usually cream) discharge from the prepuce; it frequently affects young dogs.

Treatment The basic principle is cleanliness. The penis should be exposed and bathed with a mild disinfectant. All discharge and scabs should be soaked away. Then a soothing antibiotic ointment is usually applied. This treatment should be repeated twice daily until the condition is cured. In young dogs, the condition often is self-terminating.

Where growths are present, these must be treated. Veterinary advice is essential.

See also Penis, Contagious Granuloma; Tumours.

Contagious Granuloma An infection type of 'growth' spread by sexual contact. Seen as pink or red raspberry-like lumps on the penis. Blood may be seen at the end of the penis. This condition is not usually found in Britain but is common in some warmer countries. A dog with this condition should not be used for stud. Treatment may be possible, using injections or by surgical means. Veterinary advice is essential.

As this disease is spread by sexual contact, it is sensible to arrange that all bitches that have been mated by a dog later found to be affected should be examined to determine if they are showing signs of the disease.

Discharge from, *see* Balanitis.

Erection Prolonged, *see* Paraphimosis.

Growths on, *see* Penis, Contagious Granuloma; Tumours.

Paraphimosis The condition where the penis becomes erect, protrudes from the sheath, and cannot return to the normal relaxed state without assistance.

The cause is usually that the hairs round the sheath become turned inwards and grip the penis in such a way that this condition occurs. Occasionally a dog may have a smaller opening of the sheath than usual, which produces the same effect.

Treatment Two people are needed. One should restrain the dog on its back, while the second lubricates the penis with oil (olive, salad or baby, or liquid paraffin) and then pulls the sheath backwards to relieve the pressure on the hairs and the penis. Normally the penis returns to its normal position within a few moments.

It is wrong to place ice or cold water on the distended penis.

If this condition recurs, veterinary advice should be sought.

Phimosis The inability to protrude the penis beyond the preputial opening because the latter is too small. This abnormality is practically always congenital, so the dog should not be used for breeding.

A veterinary surgeon can correct the condition by enlarging the opening surgically. This is a relatively minor operation, but care must be taken afterwards to ensure that the dog does not lick the site of the operation.

Pericarditis Inflammation of the sac that encloses the heart. This condition is not common in the dog and can be difficult for the unqualified person to detect. However, symptoms usually include rapid respiration, while the pulse is fast and weak. The dog usually has a high temperature, and there may be pain on the left side of the chest.

Periostitis

Treatment by a veterinary surgeon is essential.
Periostitis Inflammation of the membrane surrounding a bone. Usually caused by injury, infection, or the spread of inflammatory reaction from a surrounding tissue such as a tendon or ligament.

There is pain, and, where a limb is involved, lameness. The skin over the site of the trouble may be discoloured. Where infection or reaction is severe, abscesses may develop. At a later stage the bone becomes thickened but the pain is reduced.

In severe cases, the dog may have a high temperature, may not wish to move or to eat, and the blood vessels in the inflamed region may be distended and appear to throb.

Treatment must be carried out by a veterinary surgeon. Rest is essential. Temporary aid may be provided by applying warm compresses to the affected site.

Even after treatment, the thickening of the bone may remain for a long period and may never completely disappear.

Peritonitis Inflammation of the peritoneum, the membrane that lines the abdominal cavity and covers the organs within it.

Peritonitis may be *idiopathic*—not depending on another disease; *traumatic*—due to injury; or *secondary* to inflammation or infection elsewhere.

The abdomen is hard and very painful if touched. The dog's breathing is rapid, and it sometimes utters a grunt with each breath. The pulse is very quick, while the temperature may rise 2°C above the normal. The dog may vomit, does not eat but will often take water in large amounts, and collapses after a few hours if not treated.

Treatment must be carried out by a veterinary surgeon. In the meantime, relief may be provided by applying hot fomentations to the abdomen where acute pain is present, and giving the dog a small amount ($\frac{1}{4}$–1 teaspoonful) of brandy. Warmth, rest, and a restricted intake of food and water are essential.

Perspiration The dog perspires mainly from the pads of the feet, through the mouth and tongue when panting, and only very slightly through the skin.

Perthe's Disease A disease in humans affecting the articular head of the femur. The name is sometimes used to refer to hip dysplasia (q.v.) in dogs.

Pharyngitis Inflammation of the pharynx. Treat as for laryngitis (q.v.).

Poisoning

Phimosis, *see* Penis.
Phlebitis   Inflammation of a vein, a condition that is rare in the dog.
Piles, *see* Haemorrhoids.
Piroplasmosis, *see* Babesiosis.
Pleurisy   Inflammation of the pleura, the lining membrane of the chest cavity and the external surface of the lungs. This condition is caused by injury or infection, or by spread of inflammation from other parts of the body.

There is a rapid, difficult and painful respiration, a high temperature, and the dog makes grunting noises. When breathing, the dog tends to use the abdominal muscles rather than the rib region. There is pain if the ribs are touched.

Veterinary attention is essential. Warmth, rest, and a bed placed on a slope so that the dog can lie with the head and chest raised, are helpful.
Pleuro-Pneumonia   Inflammation of the pleura and lungs.
Pneumonia   Inflammation of the lungs. Causes can be infection, injury, the migration of parasites (especially in young animals), or by spread of inflammation from other parts of the body.

This condition usually shows the following symptoms. The attack starts with shivering, the temperature often rises, the dog goes off its food, is quiet, has difficulty in breathing and may grunt with each breath; the pulse is full and hard, and the chest is tender on pressure. Often, if the owner listens close to the chest, it is possible to hear a grating sound (crepitation); however, this may disappear as the condition progresses and the sounds become dull, muffled, and eventually, in certain areas, may cease altogether. At the start of the attack the dog may have a cough.

Veterinary treatment is essential. Warmth, rest, and the use of inhalants such as Vick or Friar's Balsam in hot water help while waiting for professional advice.
Poisoning   This is usually the result of the dog having *swallowed* a poison. Make *absolutely* sure that all substances that could kill or harm dogs are kept out of their reach. These include rat poisons, insecticides, cleaning substances, paint, weed-killers and, of course, any medicines or tablets for humans. A dog can also be poisoned through eating the bulbs of hyacinths, narcissus or daffodils.

The plants of poinsettia, oleander and dieffenbachia may produce illness if eaten. The seeds of ricinus, the castor oil plant, and mistletoe berries can be fatal.

Poisoning

Action to be taken. Read this section through before taking any action.

1 If a dog is thought to be showing signs of poisoning, the type of poison must be quickly identified and the veterinary surgeon contacted at once. He will in many cases advise that the dog should be made to vomit. This can be done by giving salt or mustard in water, or a crystal of washing soda (about the size of a large pea) by mouth.

2 An antidote for most *acid* poisons is bicarbonate of soda—a teaspoonful in a cup of warm water. Crushed egg shells can also be used.

For *alkali* poisons, three or four tablespoons of vinegar or lemon- or lime-juice should be given.

3 The dog should be kept warm and quiet; fresh air helps. If respiration or heart action stops, artificial respiration (q.v.) should be started.

4 If the owner does not know what poison has been swallowed, await veterinary advice. Where the poisonous agent is known, follow the appropriate instructions as listed below.

Acids   Do not induce vomiting. Act as (2) above.
Aconite   Do not induce vomiting. Give tea without milk.
Alkalis   Do not induce vomiting. Act as (2) above.
Allonal, see Barbiturates.
Ammonia   Do not induce vomiting. Wash mouth out with water, then give vinegar.
Amytal, see Barbiturates.
Antifreeze solutions   Induce vomiting.
Antimony   Give tea without milk.
Ant-killer   Induce vomiting.
Arsenic   Induce vomiting, then give milk.
Aspirin   Induce vomiting. Observe closely for 12 hours.
Atropine in drops or tablets   Induce vomiting.
Automobile polish liquid   Do not induce vomiting.
Barbiturates   Induce vomiting. Keep the dog moving.
Barium   Induce vomiting, give Epsom or Glauber's salts in water.
Belladonna, see Atropine.
Benzine   Do not induce vomiting.
Bleach   Do not induce vomiting.
Boric acid   Induce vomiting.

Poisoning

Bulbs of plants   Induce vomiting.
Camphorated oil   Induce vomiting.
Carbolic acid   Do not induce vomiting. Give egg and milk.
Carbon monoxide fumes from fires or gas   Give artificial respiration. Fresh air essential.
Carbon tetrachloride   Do not induce vomiting.
Caustic lime, potash, soda, see Lye.
Cigarettes   Induce vomiting.
Cleaning fluid   Do not induce vomiting.
Coal gas, see Carbon monoxide.
Cockroach powder   Induce vomiting.
Codeine (tablets or liquid containing)   Induce vomiting.
Contraceptive pills   Do nothing.
Copper salts   Give solution of permanganate of potash.
Cough syrups   Induce vomiting.
Cresol, see Carbolic acid.
Creosote, see Carbolic acid.
DDT   Induce vomiting.
Digitalis   Induce vomiting, then give Epsom salts and milk.
Drain cleaner, see Lye.
Dry cleaning fluid   Do not induce vomiting.
Fly poisons (if containing arsenic)   Induce vomiting, then give milk.
Fowler's solution   Induce vomiting. Give milk.
Fuel oil   Do not induce vomiting. Give milk.
Furniture polish   Do not induce vomiting. Give milk.
Gasoline   Do not induce vomiting.
Hydrochloric acid   Do not induce vomiting. Give bicarbonate of soda (a teaspoonful) in water.
Ink   Induce vomiting.
Insects   Do nothing, but observe the dog for 1 hour (symptoms of systemic upset are unlikely but possible); treat for collapse if necessary.
Insect sprays   Do not induce vomiting.
Iodine   Give bread or porridge, then induce vomiting.
Iron tablets   Induce vomiting.
Kerosene (paraffin)   Do not induce vomiting.
Lead   Induce vomiting, then give Epsom salts in water.
Lighter fuel   Do not induce vomiting.
Luminal, see Barbiturates.

Poisoning

Lye Do not induce vomiting. Wash mouth with water. Give vinegar diluted 1 part to 3 parts water, lemon-juice or grapefruit juice.
Lysol, see Carbolic acid.
Matches (now normally harmless) Do nothing, but watch the dog for 3 hours.
Metaldehyde (slug killer) Induce vomiting.
Methylated spirit Induce vomiting.
Mercury Induce vomiting, then give white of egg, milk.
Mothballs Induce vomiting.
Mouse poisons, see Rat and mouse poisons.
Mushrooms and toadstools Induce vomiting.
Nembutal, see Barbiturates.
Nicotine Induce vomiting.
Nitric acid, as for Sulphuric acid.
Paint Induce vomiting, then give Epsom salts in water.
Paraffin Do not induce vomiting.
Petrol Do not induce vomiting.
Phenobarbitone, phenobarbital, see Barbiturates.
Phenol, see Carbolic acid.
Phosphorus Induce vomiting, then give barley water. Do not give oils or fats in any form.
Plant sprays Induce vomiting.
Plants Induce vomiting.
Potash, see Lye.
Quicklime, see Lye.
Rat and mouse poisons As these can contain many different poisonous constituents, no general rule can be given. When the constituents are known, proceed as follows:
ANTU (a thiourea compound) Very rapid in action, *see* Collapse.
Arsenic Induce vomiting, then give milk.
Metaldehyde Induce vomiting.
Phosphorus Induce vomiting, then give barley water. Do not give fats or oil.
Red squill Itself causes the dog to vomit.
Thallium Induce vomiting.
Warfarin Do not feed; protect the dog from injury, however slight.
Zinc phosphide Give tea, milk, white of egg.

Santonin Induce vomiting. Give no fats or oils.
Seconal, see Barbiturates.
Shoe polish Induce vomiting.
Sleeping tablets, see Barbiturates.
Slug killer Induce vomiting.
Soda bicarbonate Will usually cause no harm.
Soda, caustic, see Lye.
Soda, washing Will usually cause vomiting; *see* Lye.
Strychnine, see Lye.
Sulphuric acid Do not induce vomiting. Wash dog's face and mouth with plenty of fresh water. Give 1 teaspoonful of bicarbonate of soda in water.
Tar products, see Carbolic acid.
Thallium preparation Induce vomiting.
Tobacco Induce vomiting.
Turpentine Induce vomiting.
Washing soda, see Lye.
Weed killers Induce vomiting.
White spirit, see Turpentine.
Wintergreen oil Induce vomiting.
Zinc salts Give teaspoonful of washing soda in warm water, tea, milk, white of egg.
Pregnancy, *see* Whelping.
Preputial Catarrh, *see* Penis, Balanitis.
Preputial Orifice too small, *see* Penis, Phimosis.
Progressive Retinal Atrophy, *see* Hereditary Abnormalities.
Prolapse, *See* Rectum; Vagina.
Prostate Gland One of the accessory sex glands. It lies at the neck of the bladder in the male dog, and partly surrounds the urethra.

ENLARGEMENT OF Common in the male dog. When enlarged, the gland interferes with the flow of urine and may obstruct the passage of a motion. Irritation may be caused to the perineal region. Diagnosis is confirmed by internal examination via the rectum.

Treatment must be undertaken by a veterinary surgeon. This may involve hormonal tablets, injections or surgery. Castration (q.v.) will usually cause the gland to diminish in size.

Protozoa One-celled animals, some of which can cause diseases in dogs. Thus coccidia and giardia infest the digestive tract, while

Pruritus Ani

piroplasma and leishmania live in the blood. The latter may also invade the liver, bone-marrow and spleen.

Pruritus Ani, *see* Anus.

Pruritus of the Skin Irritation of the skin which may occur in many conditions without visible skin lesions, and in some cases without discoverable cause. It may be associated with chronic indigestion, chronic inflammation of the kidneys, allergy, or reflex irritation from some alimentary abnormality (e.g. worms). It may accompany jaundice, diabetes and various infections.

Irritation of the skin due to external parasites, or alterations in the structure of the skin, are not included under the heading of true pruritus. Overfeeding, restricted exercise, constipation, a diet with excessive carbohydrate, old age and many other factors may predispose to the onset of this condition.

The affected animal will lick, scratch or rub the affected part and may produce a scaly or thickened condition of the skin, and sometimes even severe sores.

Treat in the same way as for eczema (q.v.).

Pseudo Diabetes The condition where the pancreas is unable to function properly, due to chronic inflammation. The digestion and water control of the body are particularly affected. The dog loses weight but the abdomen may become enlarged; it will eat and drink excessively while the motions often contain amounts of undigested fat. Veterinary advice is essential.

Pseudo Hodgkin's Disease A progressive fatal disease where tumour formation occurs in the lymph nodes (glands).

In the early stages, the enlargement of the glands causes no pain or discomfort. Later pressure of the enlarged glands may cause pain or disturbance of other organs.

There is no treatment, but the course of the condition can be delayed by drugs. Obtain veterinary advice.

Pseudo Rabies This disease is rare in the dog. If it occurs, it is fatal, usually within 48 hours. It is characterised by intense irritation of the skin, which makes the dog scratch and bite itself. There is no tendency to attack or bite other dogs or persons.

Puerperal Fever This name is occasionally used when referring to an infection of the bitch's uterus following whelping (q.v.), which enters the blood-stream.

Pulse Rate The normal pulse rate varies in the number of beats per minute, according to the size of the dog. The number is fewer

Rabies

in the larger dogs than the smaller ones; e.g. a St Bernard is about 70 times a minute, a toy dog about 100 p.m. The pulse rate tends to increase with exercise.

The dog's pulse is often irregular.

In many diseases the pulse rate is increased, although in some forms of heart disease, it may be reduced.

The pulse is always quicker in the young animal and in old age.

The best place to feel and count the pulse is inside the hind leg, where the femoral artery crosses the inside of the femur.

Puppies, Having, *see* Whelping.

Purgative Medicine Laxatives should be avoided if possible, and given only on veterinary advice. To correct constipation, give the dog increased exercise, a meal containing liver or add brown sugar to the diet.

See also Constipation.

Pyometra, *see* Uterus, Inflammation of.

Pyometritis, *see* Uterus, Inflammation of.

Pyorrhoea, *see* Gum.

Rabies A virus disease of all mammals, including man, which is spread by the saliva of an infected animal entering the body of another animal, usually by biting.

The period of incubation varies from 2 weeks to 6 months, and depends on the site of infection. The virus has to travel to the brain along a nerve from the point where it entered the body. Therefore the further from the head the bite occurred the longer the incubation period.

Symptoms are basically a change of temperament followed by a period of great excitement, and, finally, if the dog survives long enough, a period of paralysis. Temperament changes are when a quiet dog becomes aggressive, or a fierce dog becomes milder. The excitement stage is characterised by the dog attacking without fear anything that moves or makes a noise. It may run for miles. The paralytic form shows symptoms of paralysis of the lower jaw and limbs. Collapse quickly follows, and then death.

Once symptoms are seen, death occurs within a week. It is while symptoms are visible that the dog can infect other dogs, animals or humans. Any person bitten by such a dog should report to their doctor as soon as possible. The dog suspected of suffering from rabies should not be killed but should be confined in a safe area from which escape is impossible. This is necessary for

Radical Paralysis

the confirmation of the disease. Once the dog is dead, the head is sent to a laboratory for detailed examination.

Where rabies is endemic, it is usual to protect dogs by injection and to repeat this vaccination at yearly or three-year intervals depending on the vaccines used.

As this disease is fatal and can infect humans, it is essential that all control measures must be rigidly enforced and that all suspected cases be reported **immediately**. People who think they may have been in contact with a possibly rabid animal should get in touch with a doctor without delay.

Radical Paralysis, *see* Paralysis.

Ranula, *see* Cysts.

Reabsorption of Puppies A bitch that was pregnant is later found to be non-pregnant, but with no discharge from the vagina. There is some debate about the incidence of this condition.

Rectal Feeding This method of feeding is used when it is impossible for the dog to be fed normally. The lower bowel is washed out with warm water to remove faecal matter, and a ready-made nutrient broth is slowly introduced. Slow introduction is imperative, otherwise straining is induced and the food rejected. The nutrient enema must be of blood heat, very concentrated, and easily assimilated.

Feeding by intravenous injection has now superseded rectal feeding.

Rectum, Prolapse of This condition is seen most commonly in aged dogs and puppies, although it can occur at any age. It is generally the result of severe straining due to constipation, diarrhoea, or invagination of the bowel (qq.v.).

The rectum 'telescopes' within itself and the resulting sausage-shaped mass protrudes through the anus.

Treatment must start as quickly as possible, otherwise the mass may become congested and swollen, and even damaged by the dog. Without treatment, the condition tends to get worse and the size of the mass increases.

The mass hanging from the dog should be bathed in warm water to clean and soften the exposed surfaces, after which, it should be gently replaced inside the rectum. This often takes time, because of the swelling that has occurred. Then it is advisable to insert a finger into the rectum to ensure that the passage is not obstructed. The use of lubricants should be avoided if possible as, although

Rickets

they make it easier to replace the prolapse, lubrication often tends to encourage a recurrence of the condition.

The prolapsed rectum should not really be treated by the owner, but should be attended to by a veterinary surgeon, provided he can be reached within a reasonable time (2–3 hours). Should there be a further prolapse, the advice and help of a qualified person is essential.

Redness of Skin This may be due to heat, infection, allergy, parasites, or reaction to sunlight. Often commonly seen in white dogs.

Keep the dog in the shade. *See* Allergy; Eczema; Parasites, External.

Respiration, Artificial, *see* Artificial Respiration.

Rheumatism Any part of the dog can be affected by this condition. The term is often used in a general sense to refer to pain and therefore non-use or restricted use of the part concerned. Muscles, ligaments or tendons may be affected, although the term is usually limited to muscle pain. As more knowledge is gained, more conditions are recognised and the number of conditions termed 'rheumatism' decrease. It is possible that rheumatism is, in many cases, a symptom of another illness.

Mild cases often respond to rest, or to treatment with soluble aspirin (q.v.)—give 150–600 mg (according to the size of the dog) three times a day. As this drug causes some dogs to vomit, take care when giving the first dose.

Acute cases, or those that do not respond to home treatment, require veterinary attention.

Rickets A deficiency disease of young animals, characterised by the development of enlarged ends of long bones and a weakness of the shaft (mid-part) of these bones, which tends to bend.

Seen in young animals during the period of growth. The fore-legs especially tend to bow outwards. The junctions of the bones of the ribs tend to swell, and feel like a string of beads.

This condition is caused by an imbalance of the calcium and phosphorus in the diet and is aggravated by a shortage of vitamin D.

Veterinary advice is essential. To feed the dog purified bonemeal (not that which is made to be used as a horticultural fertiliser), or a supplement which has calcium and phosphorus in the proportions of 5:4 helps to prevent or correct the condition. Vitamin

Ringworm

D can be supplied by giving a teaspoonful (5 ml) of cod-liver oil once a week. *See* Section 2, 'Feeding a Dog'.
See also Achondroplasia.
Ringworm A fungus condition of the dog's skin, which may be caused by *Trichophyton*, *Microsporum*, *Oidmella* or *Oospora*.

The name is derived from the circular lesions that are sometimes seen on the skin when infection occurs. However, many cases do not show these lesions and the infestation can often be diagnosed only by examining hair samples. Veterinary treatment is essential.

Ringworm can spread to humans.
Roundworms, *see* Parasites, Internal.
Rubber Jaw, *see* Osteomalacia.
Rupture This term has various meanings. It is applied to the condition similar to a hernia, but where the lining membrane, as well as the wall of the cavity in which the organs enclosed are normally constrained, is torn.

The term may be used for the tearing across of tendons, ligaments, nerves, arteries, etc.
See also Hernia.
St Vitus's Dance, *see* Chorea.
Sarcoma, *see* Tumours.
Sarcoptic Mange, *see* Mange.
Scalds, *see* Burns and Scalds.
Sciatica This term was formerly used for the pain that might result when a dog was given an intramuscular injection. It is not the same as the term applied to humans.
Scissor Bite The term used when the teeth of the lower jaw touch the inner aspect of the upper incisors.
Sea Sickness, *see* Travel Sickness.
Season, *see* Oestrus.
Sebaceous Cyst, *see* Cysts.
Septicaemia The condition where bacteria circulate in the blood and are therefore carried to all parts of the body. The dog is obviously unwell, shivers, tends to lie in a cool quiet place. When the temperature (q.v.) is taken, this is found to be raised.

Veterinary treatment must be given at once. Antibiotics are normally used. The dog should be kept warm, and food and water offered in small amounts. If these are not taken, they should not be left in front of the dog. *See* Nursing.
Sexual Excitement Some dogs try to ride people's legs, or

soft objects, etc., and tend to lick themselves repeatedly, all of which is objectionable.

In young animals this may disappear as they become older.

Sedatives are sometimes useful (e.g. potassium bromide, 300 mg three times a day), but do not always prove effective.

In many cases the remedy is surgical castration or spaying.

Shock　A condition which may occur following injury, disease, or an operation. Fright and pain may also contribute to its development.

Shock has been defined as 'circulatory failure accompanied by depression of vital functions'. In practice, shock can be recognised by paleness of the mucous membranes, shivering, thirst, apathy and weakness, dilated pupils, and a weak but rapid pulse. There may be vomiting and a subnormal temperature.

It is essential to reassure the shocked dog by speaking calmly and gently. It should be kept warm by wrapping it in blankets. Hot-water bottles should be provided, but only gradually, as if heat is supplied too suddenly, the danger of the condition may be increased. The bottles should be just above blood heat and placed outside the blankets. As the dog recovers, the heat can be increased. Fresh air should be provided. The animal should lie so that the head is slightly lower than the hind-quarters; the head and neck should be straight.

Treat as for collapse (q.v.), if this occurs.

Veterinary attention is essential.

Note. If the shock was caused by electricity, turn off the power before starting home treatment.

Shyness　A behaviour pattern where the dog does not act naturally in the presence of humans. It may be hereditary, the result of trauma or stress, or because of incorrect management of the dog during early life. *See* Section 2, 'Canine Behaviour Patterns'.

Treatment is often difficult. Training with a qualified trainer is the most satisfactory method of correction.

Snake-Bite　If a dog is bitten by a snake, swelling occurs at the site, and the dog is in pain. The breathing becomes laboured. If the snake was truly venomous, the bite may cause paralysis, coma and death.

Open the site, and rub crystals of permanganate of potash into the wound. Tie a tourniquet (q.v.) if possible between the bite and the trunk of the body. Keep the dog quiet and warm.

Snoring

Snoring Any dog may snore, but this is particularly common in the short-nosed breeds. It is not normally a sign of ill-health. The only treatment is to try to ensure that when the dog is asleep the head and neck are straight.

For overweight dogs, slimming will often stop this habit.

Snorting A noise and action that seem to imply that the dog is trying to remove some obstruction from the nose. It may often be noticed when the dog enters an area where the temperature is in marked contrast to the previous position; e.g. when it leaves a warm house and goes out into cold air.

Although this may be due to infection or disease, it is commonly a sign that catarrh exists in the nasal passages. Very occasionally the condition may be caused by a polypus in the nasal passages or by worms.

The treatment is not always easy. If the cause can be found, this must be treated. If not, inhalation of Vick or Friar's Balsam will often relieve the condition. Otherwise, veterinary treatment is required.

Sore Throat, *see* Laryngitis; Pharyngitis.

Spaying The rendering of the female dog sterile by an operation to remove the ovaries and uterus. Although a major operation, it has become routine in all good veterinary practices and is one that can be considered by the owner to be without too much risk. As with all operations, an element of danger exists, but this is small.

The result is that the bitch does not have seasons, false pregnancies, pyometra or pyometritis. It is generally considered that this operation is ideal for a bitch from which the owner does not wish to breed.

Sprains The damage to muscles, ligaments, or tendons, due to trauma. The condition often resolves without treatment, provided that the injury is not aggravated by too much activity. Therefore rest is essential. Veterinary treatment is advisable, and is required if the dog's response to rest is not good. Veterinary treatment is often said to be essential for all sprains or muscular pain.

Squint, *see* Eye.

Sterility The inability of an animal to propagate the species. There may be many causes.

In the *male*, it may be due to castration, deformity of the penis, injury, deformity of the testes or any of the sexual organs, lack of sexual drive, etc.

Stomach Tube

In the *female*, it may result from spaying, deformity of the sexual organs, etc., but most commonly from an unusual, but normal, time of ovulation (*see* Oestrus). This occurs where the bitch releases the eggs (ovulation) at an unexpected time. If this is suspected, she should be tested each morning during her season using Tes-Tape (Eli Lilly, Basingstoke). This is a small piece of tape that is placed in the vagina for two seconds and then removed. At the start of the season, the tape does not change colour. Later, it will suddenly change to green, which indicates that glucose is present in the discharge. The ideal time for mating should be 24 hours after this colour change is first seen.

The advice of a veterinary surgeon is essential.

The general condition of a dog of either sex must be considered. An unhealthy, under-exercised, or over-weight animal is unlikely to have the sexual power of the fit one.

Stifle Joint, injury to This joint corresponds to the knee joint in man, and is very prone to injury in the dog. All weaknesses believed to relate to the articular surface of this region require veterinary attention.

Stings Following a sting, the part attacked usually swells.

Where the causal insect is not known, the sting, if present, should be removed and the area bathed in vinegar.

Where the mouth is involved, the sting, if present, should be removed, and the whole mouth washed with a solution of bicarbonate of soda.

If the dog appears extremely unwell or has not recovered within half an hour, a veterinary surgeon should be consulted.

See also Snake-Bite.

BEE-STINGS These are common in the dog, usually on the head or around the lips. If possible, the sting should be removed using forceps or the finger-nail; scratch it out rather than pull, to avoid the possibility that more of the poison is forced into the tissue. The area should be washed with a solution of bicarbonate of soda (5 g in 100 ml water). Alternatively, the powder itself can be applied to the sting wound.

If marked swelling occurs, veterinary advice should be sought.

WASP-STINGS Apply vinegar.

Stomach Tube An instrument used to place substances within the stomach without the aid of the animal.

Used in very young dogs when hand reared. This has the

Stoutness

advantage of speed for the owner but has the disadvantage that in inexperienced hands the life of the puppy may be endangered.

Stoutness, *see* Obesity.

Stroke The condition of unconsciousness, or partial unconsciousness, due to haemorrhage into the substance of the brain, or of clotting of blood in the cerebral blood vessels. Strokes are seen mainly in older dogs.

The attack is very rapid. Vomiting may occur. The degree of loss of consciousness varies. If the dog is able to stand, the head is often held to one side. The animal is distressed and in many cases the eyes show a wavering movement where they move fairly rapidly from side to side.

The dog should be kept as quiet as possible, and placed in a darkened room. No stimulants of any kind should be given. Water in small amounts may be supplied.

Veterinary attention is essential.

Stye, *see* Eyelid.

Subnormal Temperature, *see* Collapse; Haemorrhage, Internal; Shock.

Suffocation, *see* Asphyxia.

Sunstroke, *see* Heat-Stroke.

Swimmers Puppies born suffering from achondroplasia (q.v.). The name is given because the puppies resemble human swimmers doing the breast-stroke.

Synovitis Inflammation of a joint, usually caused by injury, infection, or the spread of inflammation from adjoining areas. In most cases there is pain and lameness.

Veterinary advice is essential.

The joint may be bathed alternately with hot and cold water, and the dog given soluble aspirin (q.v.) (150–600 mg, depending on size) to relieve the discomfort while waiting for expert advice.

Tail, Docking of The removal of part of the tail for aesthetic reasons. This is usually carried out when the puppy is 3 to 5 days old and causes little suffering. However, there is no advantage to the dog if this is done and many people consider that unnecessary operations of this nature should be avoided.

For pedigree dogs that are to be sent to countries where this docking is accepted, it is probably better to perform this operation at an early age rather than later, when the effects on the dog are more severe.

Teeth

Different breeds require that the tail be docked to differing lengths. The Fox Terrier should have three-fifths of the tail left; Irish and Airedale Terriers rather less than half; Spaniels, about two-fifths; Griffons, about one-third.

The breeds that may be docked according to the Kennel Club Rules are Spaniels (except Irish Water), Airedale Terriers, Fox Terriers, Irish Terriers, Kerry Blue Terriers, Sealyham Terriers, Welsh Terriers, Old English Sheepdogs, Poodles, Schipperkes, Schnauzers, Griffon Bruxellois, Toy Spaniels, Yorkshire Terriers, and other breeds that the committee 'may from time to time determine'.

Tail, Sores on Tip, *see* Haemorrhage, Tail.

Tapeworm, *see* Parasites, Internal.

Teats, Sore This condition may occur when a bitch is feeding her puppies. The teat becomes swollen and the skin develops cracks and becomes hardened.

If possible, the puppies should be encouraged to feed from other milk glands for part of the day. The teat should be cleaned and dressed with boracic cream.

If the milk gland becomes hardened, treat as for mastitis (q.v.).

TEETH

Each tooth is divided into three parts. The part visible when looking into the mouth is the *crown*; below this is the *neck*, the constricted part encircled by the gum, which divides the crown from the *root*, which is inserted into a cavity (the alveolus) in the jaw bone.

Each tooth is made up of three different structures. The external layer, or enamel, which gives the tooth its white appearance, consists of a thin layer and covers the crown only. Immediately underneath the enamel is situated the dentine, which comprises most of the tooth. In the middle is a foramen, or small cavity, containing the pulp, which consists of a membrane, nerve and small blood-vessels to supply nourishment, etc. to the tooth.

See also Dentition.

Care of It is sensible to examine the teeth of a dog once a week, bearing the following points in mind.

The puppy. Are the teeth coming through the gums? If so, are these sore? Is there enough space for the erupting teeth? Are the adult teeth appearing before the temporary ones have been shed?

Teeth

The adult.   Are the teeth discoloured or marked in any way? Is scale developing? Are any teeth loose?

Naturally, if any defect is thought to exist this must have attention.

Routine cleaning of the teeth is a sound idea and one that the dog will accept, provided that it is commenced at an early age. Toothpaste can be used—if it contains fluoride, so much the better, as this tends to strengthen the teeth.

Caries   Decay of part of the surface of the tooth. This can be seen as dark marks or as holes in the teeth. *See also* Breath, Foul.

Treatment consists in cleaning the area and filling the cavity, or the tooth may have to be extracted. Treatment must be carried out by a veterinary surgeon.

The condition appears to occur most commonly when a dog's diet is lacking in hard matter which requires chewing.

Dental Fistula   An abscess formation which usually appears below the eye and which may rupture and continue to discharge if left untreated. It is usually caused by infection of the root of the 4th upper premolar tooth. Treatment normally consists of the removal of this tooth under a general anaesthetic. Recovery is usually complete. This condition is often called a *molar abscess*.

Dentition   A normal adult dog has 42 teeth—20 in the upper jaw, 22 in the lower. The 6 front teeth in both the upper and lower jaw are called incisors. Behind these are the canines, one on each side of both jaws. The premolars and molars are the big grinding teeth at the back of the jaw; 4 premolars and 2 molars in the upper jaw; 4 premolars and 3 molars in the lower.

At birth the puppy has no teeth. Later temporary or milk teeth appear. From 3–4 weeks the incisors erupt, the temporary canines appearing at about the same time, while the three temporary premolars follow at about 6–9 weeks. The time of eruption of the temporary teeth varies very considerably.

The permanent teeth, as they appear, push out the temporary teeth; the incisors at about 14 to 16 weeks of age, the canines about two weeks later, and the premolars at about 5–8 months. Again, the age is very variable.

Where the permanent teeth do not force away the temporary teeth, these may remain in the jaw and cause trouble. In some cases they have to be removed under a general anaesthetic to provide space for the developing permanent teeth.

Temperature, Taking

Erosion of Enamel This is seen when a dog had some form of physical upset at the time that the tooth enamel was being formed. At one time, this was called *distemper teeth*, as teeth of dogs recovering from an attack of distemper at 2 to 3 months of age often showed this condition.

A discoloured area is visible on the tooth or teeth (usually more than one is affected). There is no treatment, but the existence of the condition means that the dog's teeth are weaker than normal, and the teeth and gums are more likely to become unhealthy as the dog ages.

Scale on The formation of scale (or tartar) on the teeth is common in the dog, particularly those who are fed with soft food. Scale can be seen as hard crusts on the teeth just above the line of the gums, between the teeth and on the inner side of the front incisor teeth.

If not treated, the condition becomes progressively worse: the teeth become loosened, the gums recede, infection and ulceration of the gums may develop and a bad mouth odour is noticeable.

Treatment consists of removing the scale, usually under a general anaesthetic. The chewing of hard biscuits may assist in the mild case. It is essential that treatment is carried out at an early stage to ensure that no permanent damage develops. Once a dog has this condition it is likely that the condition will recur after treatment, so the mouth should be regularly examined for further signs of scale.

Tartar on, *see* Scale on.

Telling Dog's Age by Not a very accurate method of assessment. It must be remembered that all dogs are individuals, and that the larger ones tend to erupt their teeth earlier than the smaller breeds.

See also Age, How to Determine; Teeth, Dentition.

Toothache This is usually due to the formation of scale and degeneration of the tooth roots. A molar abscess often develops if the 4th upper premolar tooth is infected (*see* Dental Fistula).

Veterinary attention is needed. Temporary relief can be provided by giving 300–600 mg soluble aspirin, depending on size of the dog, and bathing the mouth with a solution of common salt.

See also Abscess; Teeth, Scale on.

Temperature, Taking, *see* Section 4.

Testicles, Enlargement of This condition can be due to injury, haemorrhage or tumour formation and is most commonly seen in older dogs. It should not be confused with scrotal hernia (*see* Hernia, Inguinal).

Veterinary treatment is required. Rest is useful. When a tumour has formed, it is often necessary to remove the testicle concerned.

Testicles, Inflammation of, *see* Orchitis.

Tetanus This disease is extremely rare in the dog, as most have a natural immunity.

Dogs suffering from tetanus tend to stand stiff and still with the jaws shut. Violent spasms may occur.

The affected dog should be placed in a cool, darkened room away from noise. A veterinary surgeon should be called at once.

Thermometer The instrument used to measure body temperature (q.v.).

Thirst The desire to drink. If excessive, it may be due to gastritis, chronic kidney disease, diarrhoea, diabetes, etc. (qq.v.). Whatever the cause, there is usually loss of weight, wastage of muscles and enlargement of the abdomen.

Treatment must depend on the cause. Veterinary advice is essential. Water should be provided until advice is obtained but the amount offered should be regulated. 'Little and often' is the ideal.

Throat, Sore The dog may have difficulty in swallowing, barking or drinking. The lymph nodes (glands) at the angle of the lower jaw are usually swollen.

A sore throat may be a localised condition or part of a generalised infection.

Treat as for laryngitis (q.v.) and seek veterinary advice.

Ticks These are external parasites, often also to be found on sheep and hedgehogs. Those infesting dogs are usually of the *Ixodes* species. They are small when they first become attached to a dog but rapidly grow until they look like a grey bean about 0·5 cm in length. They may carry infection.

A dog infested with ticks should be bathed or powdered as for fleas (q.v.).

Tie So called because when dogs mate, the sphincter muscles in the female hold the penis of the male so that the two cannot separate for a period. This period usually lasts for 2 to 20 minutes, during which time it is dangerous to try to separate the animals. Given time, they will separate naturally.

TONGUE

Black This is a sign of a deficiency disease, the symptoms of which resemble those of one form of leptospirosis (q.v.). It is directly due to a deficiency of vitamin B2 and is treated by the injection of massive doses of that vitamin.

Inflammation of This is usually noticed as the tongue is swollen and red and tends to hang out of the mouth. It is often caused by a bite or sting, or following infection of the gums due to tooth trouble.

The cause must be determined and treated, and the mouth should be washed with warm water. Ulcers or sores should be dressed with hydrogen peroxide (10 vol.). This will cause frothing where it is applied, but it cleans and reduces infection.

Recovery is usually very rapid (about 24 hours). Where the condition is severe, or the dog does not appear to be recovering, veterinary advice should be obtained.

Warts on These are small greyish lumps which appear on the surface of the tongue, and may also occur on the gums, cheeks and lips. They are usually seen in puppies, where they can occur in great numbers and may interfere with eating. A dirty-looking saliva may dribble from the mouth. They are contagious from one puppy to another, so that affected puppies should be isolated.

Veterinary advice is needed. The dog's mouth may be washed out with a teaspoonful of bicarbonate of soda dissolved in 0·25 litres of warm water. The warts should not be cut.

Wounds and Ulcers on These may be caused by the dog biting the tongue, by ulceration spreading from other parts of the mouth, or by the spread of infection from other parts of the body. They may also be associated with misplaced or broken teeth, scale on the teeth, or other mechanical defects of the mouth.

Healing normally occurs quickly. The mouth should be washed out with a teaspoonful of bicarbonate of soda in 0·25 litres of warm water.

Veterinary treatment is always advisable. If the tip or other part of the tongue becomes grey-white in colour, and appears harder than normal, veterinary advice is essential.

Tonsillitis, *see* Pharyngitis.
Toothache, *see* Teeth.

Tourniquet

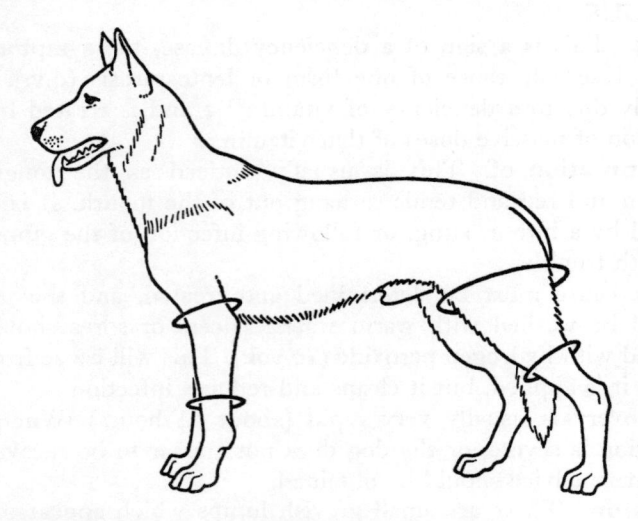

Figure 3 Places where tourniquets can be applied

Tourniquet A method of controlling haemorrhage by pressure above the point of bleeding which can be applied by a cord, tape or bandage. It is used on limbs or the tail. The tape used may be anything that is available (a tie, a dog's lead, a belt, etc.). It is placed nearer the heart than the point of bleeding. The positions where it can be applied are shown in Figure 3.

If a tourniquet has to be kept in place for any length of time, it should be eased every 3 or 4 minutes to ensure that blood circulates through the tissues and permanent damage is thus avoided.

Travel Sickness Some dogs vomit when being transported. This may be accompanied with excessive salivation and fear. A dog that is known to act in this way should not be fed or given water for 4 hours before a journey. During the journey it should be kept warm, provided with fresh air, and allowed, if possible, to see and hear its owner. Travel sickness tablets made for children are often of help; the dose should be adjusted to the size of the dog. Sedative tablets are usually effective but should be used only after veterinary advice has been obtained.

Trichiasis, *see* Eyelashes, Ingrowing.

Tuberculosis A disease caused by the bacterium *Mycobacterium* *tuberculosis*, which can occur in man and most animals, but is now rare in the dog. When it is diagnosed in a dog, it has usually been caught from direct contact from a human with the disease or from contaminated milk or meat.

Symptoms are very variable and depend on the site of the infection within the dog.

Treatment by a veterinary surgeon is essential. Fresh air and good food aid recovery. However, since a dog can spread the infection to a human being, this is a factor which may influence the decision to treat or destroy the dog.

TUMOURS
These are the result of an abnormal development of cells within the body. Their growth does not conform with the laws of tissue growth, and these new growths are parasitic on the body where they are growing.

Tumours are relatively common in the dog. They can be separated into many different types, but for the purpose of this book may be divided into *benign* and *malignant tumours*.

BENIGN TUMOURS These usually grow slowly, and are restricted to the point where they first develop. They may press on surrounding tissues but do not invade the neighbouring areas. They are usually enclosed in a capsule. If completely removed, they do not recur.

MALIGNANT TUMOURS These usually grow rapidly, spread to neighbouring tissues, and can develop in other parts of the body by being carried in the circulation. Because of this, surgical removal rarely completely removes the cancerous development. Malignant tumours, if near the surface of the body, may ulcerate through the skin.

Tumours may develop in any part of the body. Most require surgical treatment, if this is at all possible, but some respond to treatment by drugs or hormones. Veterinary treatment is essential and should be started as early as possible.

There is a tendency on the part of some owners to delay the first veterinary consultation, as they are afraid of being told that the condition is incurable. This is, in fact, bad reasoning, as the earlier the condition is diagnosed the more chance is there of a recovery.

The above paragraph is extremely important. Early treatment is essential, as some benign tumours may eventually become

Ulcers

malignant. Surgical removal of a growth is easier, and has fewer after-effects if it is carried out when the growth is small.
See also Cysts.

Mammary Tumours in the mammary glands (the milk-producing glands) are common in the bitch. They can be felt as hard lumps and may occur singly or in several places. Very occasionally they may feel soft, but this is the result of inflammation or infection within the tumour.

It is essential that these tumours be treated as early as possible. Most are benign and do not recur after surgical removal.

Treatment consists of surgical removal, or control by supplying certain drugs in small amounts over a long period. These are usually supplied in the form of a pellet which is placed under the skin, after a local anaesthetic. It must be stressed that drugs are not always successful, and that even when such treatment does prove effective, the tumour is controlled, not removed, so that there is always the possibility of recurrence.

Tumours that are left untreated may not grow beyond a certain size, but there is always a danger that they may spread to other parts of the body, become infected or ulcerated, or cause discomfort to the dog. Veterinary advice is therefore always required.

Ulcers For the purpose of treatment, ulcers may be divided into internal ulcers and those occurring on the skin.

INTERNAL ULCERS These are usually diagnosed after a detailed examination by the veterinary surgeon, and professional advice is essential. If the digestive tract is involved, food and slightly warm water should be given frequently in small amounts. The food should be bland (soft), and without strong flavours or excessive salt.

ULCERS OF THE SKIN These should be cleaned with warm water and then dried gently and dressed with a soothing ointment or acriflavine emulsion. If possible, the sore should not be covered. However, it is essential that the dog does not lick or scratch the site; bandaging may be required to prevent this. If the sore does not heal, obtain the advice of a veterinary surgeon.

Where ulceration develops because of some other condition, this other condition must be treated.

Undershot Jaw, *see* Jaw.

Uraemia This condition develops when, because the kidney,

Urine, Sediment in

or another part of the body that affects the kidney, is diseased, the toxic materials within the body that the kidneys should excrete are retained within the body, and circulate in the blood-stream.

The dog will usually have a bad mouth odour.

This condition can be extremely serious, as the dog loses its appetite. There may be constipation, giddiness and vomiting. It becomes sleepy, and the temperature often rises. At a later stage the temperature drops to below normal; there may be abdominal pain, with vomiting and diarrhoea. Convulsions follow. The white of the eyes are usually blood-shot. The urine is dark in colour.

Treatment depends on the cause. Veterinary advice is essential. If the dog can drink without being sick, water should be provided in small amounts at frequent intervals until expert help is obtained.

Urethritis Inflammation of the urethra. This condition is more common in the male. The usual cause is localised infection, which is increased in many cases by the passage of urinary stones.

Treatment by a veterinary surgeon is essential, and the dog should be encouraged to drink. If professional treatment is delayed, hexamine (150–600 mg, depending on the size of the dog) may be given 3 times a day.

Urinary Incontinence The involuntary passing of urine. The condition occurs most often in young dogs, especially females, and especially when the dog is excited.

Normally, urinary incontinence is due to poor muscular strength of the sphincter muscles of the bladder, to nervous stress arising from improper upbringing, or to some factor, often of genetic origin, that predisposes to this condition.

In older dogs, the cause may be inflammation of the bladder or its sphincter, sometimes enlargement of the prostate gland or the development of urinary calculi.

Veterinary advice is essential.

Urine, Sediment in The dog's urine may be discoloured, white and cloudy, or clear, but of a high colour. When it is cold, there is a thick, yellowish-white deposit.

If the dog is already sick, with a high temperature, this sediment becomes a symptom rather than a condition, and no specific treatment is required as the treatment of the existing illness should make it clear up. Otherwise it is essential to find the type of salt being excreted and a urine sample (q.v.) should be taken. Veterinary advice is needed.

Urine Sample (Specimen)

As a first aid measure, the dog should be encouraged to drink, bicarbonate of soda should be added to the water (a teaspoonful to 0·25 litres), and the diet should not contain red meat.

Urine Sample (Specimen), how to take It can be collected as it is passed, in a pan or bottle; or on a sheet of plastic placed on the ground where the dog habitually urinates; or with a catheter. A catheter should be used only by an expert—sterile conditions and great care are the primary considerations.

Urticaria An allergic condition of the skin, where raised areas appear (*see* Allergy).

Uterine Inertia The condition where, at the time of whelping, the muscles of the uterus are unable to contract. It may be *primary*, because of some physical inability of the bitch, or *secondary*, where it is caused by tiredness or some other condition.

UTERUS

Inflammation of This occurs more often in the older bitch, and usually within the first few weeks after a season.

The condition can take several forms, and descriptive names can be confusing to the ordinary dog-owner. In this book the condition is considered to be of two types: *pyometra* and *pyometritis*.

PYOMETRA Inflammation of the uterus, where pus or fluid collects within it. This condition is usually due to a hormonal imbalance, and is more common in bitches that have not produced puppies. In an 'open pyometra', the fluid is able to flow away from the bitch as a vaginal discharge because the cervix is relaxed; in a 'closed pyometra', the discharge is unable to flow away as the cervix is closed. The latter is the more serious.

This condition must be treated by a veterinary surgeon.

PYOMETRITIS This is caused by infection. There is usually a heavy discharge from the vagina and vulva. The bitch is off her food, listless, and drinks slightly more than normal. She may vomit. The temperature is raised.

Veterinary treatment is essential.

Inflammation of the uterus (metritis) can also occur when an afterbirth is retained (*see* Whelping).

In general, all conditions of this nature are serious. If a discharge is visible, the bitch is less ill than if the collection of liquid is retained within the uterus. If the condition has been developing for some weeks or longer, the owner often notices that the dog has suddenly appeared to age.

All conditions involving the uterus must be treated by a veterinary surgeon. It is unwise to breed from a bitch that has suffered from any of these conditions, and advice should be sought on this point.

Vaccines These are products that are injected or otherwise given to produce immunity against a specific disease. They may be made from live, attenuated (weakened), or killed organisms and are normally used to prevent disease (*see* Immunity).

As vaccines rely for their action on the reaction they produce in the dog's body, there is a delay between the time they are given and that when resistance is developed.

In the dog, vaccines are commonly used against the following diseases.

DISTEMPER AND HARD PAD Booster injections are usually required every second year.

VIRAL HEPATITIS Depending on the type of vaccine used, booster injections are required each year or not at all.

LEPTOSPIROSIS Booster injections are required yearly.

RABIES Booster injections are required, but the time between each depends on the type of vaccine used.

A modified *measles* vaccine is sometimes used to protect dogs against distemper.

Vaccines are safe and reliable. It is rare that a reaction occurs, but if it does, the veterinary surgeon should be contacted at once.

In the normal way, vaccines should be given only to healthy dogs.

VAGINA
Discharge from (*see also* Uterus, Inflammation of, Pyometra). This may be caused by inflammation of the uterus, but it can occur as a slight white discharge seen just before a season commences, or after whelping (q.v.); it may be due to tumour formation, infection, etc.

Veterinary attention is essential for all the above, except for the discharge that occurs within a few days of the start of a season. In this case, as long as the bitch is fit, the only attention required is to ensure that the vagina and the external surrounding areas are kept clean.

Injuries to These are rare in the bitch and are usually seen after whelping (q.v.).

Vaginitis

Polypus of A pear-shaped growth of which the narrow end is attached to the membrane of the vagina. If one is present, the bitch frequently strains to pass water; she is seen to be constantly licking the area and may have some mucous discharge. At times, especially when she comes into season, the growth may be seen protruding through the vulva.

Treatment is by surgical removal under an anaesthetic. In a few cases, it is possible to ligate the 'stalk', using a silk or catgut thread, but this may not completely remove the growth, in which case it will recur.

Prolapse of This occasionally occurs in bitches after a season or after whelping. The prolapse is seen as a pinkish lump protruding from the vulva. This condition should not be confused with a vaginal polypus.

If not treated immediately, the part exposed becomes ulcerated.

Veterinary attention is essential.

Stricture of This condition is seen more commonly in the smaller breeds. It causes no inconvenience, and is usually discovered when a bitch is mated, when it is found that she cannot be properly covered by the male. The cause is a form of fibrous ring that prevents the dilatation of the vagina.

Treatment consists of stretching the constricted part. Although this can be done with a finger, it is essential to consult a veterinary surgeon in case other conditions are also present. Strict attention must be paid to cleanliness. There is no objection to mating the bitch immediately after this manipulation has been carried out.

Tumours of, *see* Tumours.

Vaginitis Inflammation of the vagina. When this is present, it is usually related to another condition affecting the reproductive or excretory organs. It is sensible to seek veterinary advice.

Valvular Disease, *see* Heart Disease.

Venereal Disease There are few diseases that are spread during mating in the dog. *Venereal granulomata* are growths that are common in certain parts of the world and are transmitted in this way.

See also Penis, Contagious Granuloma.

Vertigo A term formerly used to describe the 'giddy turns' that are now known to be due to heart conditions in old dogs. *See* Heart Attack.

Weighing a Dog

Vitamins, *see* Section 2, 'Canine Nutrition'.
Voice, Loss of This can be caused by pharyngitis, laryngitis (qq.v.), infection, tumours, etc. But the commonest cause is excessive barking, often when a dog is boarded.
The condition normally corrects itself within a few days.
Vomiting Dogs vomit easily and quickly. This may be due to habit, or as a symptom of illness. The latter may include indigestion, gastritis, kidney disease, peritonitis, enteritis, inflammation of the uterus, a foreign body in the stomach or intestine, liver disturbance, poisoning, etc.

The treatment depends on the cause. Food should be withheld for 24 hours. Water to drink in small amounts is good provided that it can be retained, in which case this should be offered every hour. Boiled water is better than unboiled.

A mixture of equal quantities of beaten white of egg, glucose and brandy can be given—a teaspoonful every quarter of an hour.

When the dog begins to improve and the vomiting ceases, it is advisable to feed small meals only; these should be extremely bland—baby foods or predigested preparations are ideal. Milk is not good at first as it tends to become 'heavy' when in the stomach.

Warmth, rest and quiet are essential.

Where severe vomiting occurs, or where response to home treatment is not successful, veterinary advice is essential.
Warts These are seen on all types of dogs, especially the aged.

Where the wart has a narrow neck, it is best removed by tying a ligature of silk round this narrowest part. The wart drops off after about a week. Other warts are best removed by surgery.

If a dog has a very large number of warts, these methods of control are not practical. In some cases a series of injections proves helpful.

Puppies may be found to have a form of wart which is produced by a virus; this type disappears within a few months without treatment, provided that other infection does not occur.
See also Tongue, Warts on.
Wasp Stings, *see* Stings.
Weaning, *see* Hand-Rearing of Puppies; Whelping; Section 2, 'Feeding a Dog'.
Weighing a Dog Small dogs can be weighed on ordinary household scales.

You can weigh larger dogs by using scales made for weighing

Whelping

humans. Weigh yourself, then pick up the dog and weigh yourself holding the dog. The difference between these two weights is the weight of the dog.

For a very large dog that cannot be picked up, you may be able to arrange that the dog walks onto a large parcel-weighing machine at a railway station or factory.

WHELPING (*see also* Mating; Sterility; Tie)
This term means, strictly, the birth of puppies. However, many aspects of pregnancy and post-natal care will be included in this section.

Duration of Pregnancy The gestation period in the dog is 63 days, but it can vary slightly. Provided that the bitch is well, and she has no discharge, it is not important if she carries her puppies 3 days longer than expected. If she goes longer still, then consult a veterinary surgeon.

Examination for Pregnancy There are no laboratory aids for pregnancy diagnosis in the bitch.

Between the 23rd and 27th day it is usually possible to feel the developing puppies in the abdomen. They feel like a line of marbles, each about 1 cm in diameter. To feel these, the bitch should be stood on a firm surface and held quietly by someone familiar, and be made to relax. A person standing behind her feels the abdomen with a hand on either side of the flank. The hands should exert gentle pressure until the finger-tips can feel the internal organs. The fingers are then moved slowly to search for developing puppies.

At 4 to 5 weeks the abdomen usually begins to enlarge.

At 6 weeks the mammary glands begin to swell.

By 7 to 8 weeks it is usually possible to see the puppies moving when the bitch is lying in a relaxed position.

Apart from these signs, the bitch usually undergoes a change in behaviour by becoming quieter and by eating more. However, this can also occur with a false pregnancy (q.v.), and so cannot by itself be considered as a reliable guide to pregnancy. X-rays can be used to confirm pregnancy during the last 3 weeks.

Attention during Pregnancy Any bitch must be fit before being mated, and therefore should have been taking exercise daily, continuing this throughout pregnancy and reducing the amount only when she becomes heavy during the last third of the time.

Food should be given normally for the first 5 weeks and then the

Whelping

amount gradually increased. It may be necessary to double the amount given by the 9th week, but care is essential to prevent the bitch from becoming overweight.

It is sensible to treat a bitch for roundworms when she is about 4 weeks pregnant.

Preparation for Whelping About a week before the puppies are due, the bitch should be encouraged to sleep in the place provided for her whelping. This may be a box, or basket, or even a clear area of a room. The essential points about the whelping area are:

1 There must be enough room for the bitch to lie fully extended.
2 The area must be so arranged that it is possible to examine the bitch without disturbing her.
3 There must be no draughts.
4 It must be warm, dry and light.
5 There should be some form of heating. This can be an infrared lamp (hung at the correct height above the back of the bitch), hot water bottles (which must be refilled frequently), or a dog bed specially designed with a heating element built into the structure to supply heat without any risk of damage to the dog.
6 Where a box, crate or bed is used it should be fitted with rails about 5 cm (2 inches) above the floor on the inside of the sides. These rails project away from the edges and form a safety area where a puppy can lie without being crushed if the bitch rolls.
7 For the whelping, it is sensible to provide some form of absorbant, disposable paper as a bedding material, as this is easy to clear away afterwards—newspaper is ideal.

The Whelping This is most easily described if it is considered to take place in four stages.

STAGE 1 This first stage starts when the milk glands become suddenly more enlarged, the vulva shows a mucous discharge, the bitch seeks her bed and her temperature falls to about 37·5°C (99°F).

Internally, the cervix begins to relax and the mucous plug liquefies, producing a sticky discharge. Uterine contractions start but are slight—they cause a change in the position of the membranes of the first puppy to be born.

STAGE 2 The cervix dilates; the liquefaction of the cervical plug continues and the breakdown products form a lubricating liquid; the vagina and vulva enlarge.

Whelping

Contractions are at this stage irregular and act on that part of the uterus which contains the puppy that is to be born first. If the hand is placed on the abdomen when the bitch is lying relaxed, the contractions can just be felt.

Stage 1 lasts for a very variable time; stage 2, for 3–6 hours, although it is not necessarily ominous if it is prolonged for 24 hours.

STAGE 3 The contractions become regular, and each time they occur, the abdominal muscles are seen to be moved; the bitch holds her breath each time, and pants between each strain. The first membranes (water bag) break and the liquid, which is clear but slippery, runs away. The second membrane (water bag) usually appears at the vulva, ruptures with the fluid contained running away, and the puppy's head is visible. The puppy is then produced very quickly.

STAGE 4 After the birth of the puppy, the bitch has a slight rest and then strains and produces the afterbirth (the remains of the membranes, etc. that held and maintained the puppy while it was within the uterus).

At the same time, the uterus starts to contract around the next puppy to be born. Stages 3 and 4 are then repeated for this puppy.

Stage 3 usually lasts ½ to 2 hours, and stage 4 about 5 minutes. Puppies are normally born at 15- to 30-minute intervals.

When all the puppies are born, the uterine contractions cease. The discharge (often green) continues for a variable period but may last as long as three weeks.

The above outline of the normal whelping process must be considered with the following facts in mind:

—Every bitch is an individual, and will vary in some way from every other bitch when whelping.

—The times mentioned are not exact but merely a guide.

—A puppy may be born facing backwards so that the tail end comes out of the vulva first. This is the so-called *posterior presentation*. When this happens, it is advisable to ensure that the birth is rapidly completed. (*See* later entry in this section 'How to Help'.)

—The bitch who has not produced puppies previously does not understand what is happening. The first puppy produced should be drawn to her attention if she does not realise that it has arrived.

Whelping

—Where a large litter is being produced, the time intervals between puppies may become progressively longer. This applies if there is a large number of puppies, or if the puppies are large.

Equipment Required by Owner The normal whelping requires no assistance from the owner. However, it is sensible to be prepared in case help has to be given.

The following are all that it is essential to have at hand: Rough towels, cotton wool, a mild disinfectant, scissors.

How to Help

1 Leave the bitch alone. Do nothing unless it is necessary, but keep an eye on her to make sure that if help is required, you are there to give it.

2 If things are going slowly, offer warm milk. This internal warmth often aids contractions.

3 If a puppy is half born so that one end is hanging out and becomes lodged, help should be given. Where the head is clear and the nose unblocked, help can be delayed for 2 or 3 minutes; if the tail end is visible, give assistance quickly, otherwise the puppy will suffocate when it tries to breathe.

The puppy should be grasped using a rough towel and a *gentle* pull exerted downwards and forwards, so that it is gradually pulled between the bitch's hind legs. The gentle pull is *not* to pull the puppy out of the bitch but to prevent it from returning to its original position after the bitch has moved it further out while straining. In other words, when the bitch strains, the puppy moves further out and your pull is to hold it there until the next contraction pushes the puppy still further. The whole process is usually over quickly with this help.

4 Where the puppy is born but is still attached to the afterbirth by the cord, this may be cut if the bitch does not lick the puppy. The cutting of the cord should be delayed for 2 minutes after birth to allow the blood in the membranes to enter the puppy. The cut is made as far away from the puppy as possible and should be done without pulling on the cord. A blunt pair of scissors are best (sharp ones tend to encourage bleeding).

5 The afterbirths should be removed to prevent the bitch from swallowing them.

6 If any puppy has membranes over the head, these should be removed as quickly as possible.

7 If a puppy is weak or not breathing, wipe out its mouth to

Whelping

remove liquid and rub it with a hard towel to stimulate respiration and heart action.

When to Contact your Veterinary Surgeon
Before the event, to tell him that the bitch is due to whelp and the expected date.

If the bitch becomes over-excited or hysterical.

If she is overdue by 3 days.

If she has been straining for 2 hours without producing a puppy.

If she has started to whelp but has stopped straining for more than 1 hour.

If there is bleeding which is flowing in a steady trickle.

If she collapses.

OR IF YOU ARE WORRIED.

It is better to make an unnecessary call than not to obtain veterinary advice and run the risk of losing the bitch or the puppies. When trouble occurs, it is usually more sensible to phone the veterinary surgeon and take the bitch to his surgery or clinic than to ask him to come to your house.

Caesarean Section ('Caesar')   This is a routine operation carried out by a veterinary surgeon when it is found that a bitch is unable to produce her young by normal whelping. The unborn puppies are surgically removed by opening the bitch's abdominal wall and uterus, and then suturing the incision.

The fact that a bitch has undergone such an operation does not necessarily mean that she must not be allowed to breed again. However, expert advice on this point must always be obtained.

After Whelping   There is usually a dark green mucous discharge which oftens turns pink after 13 hours.

After about 6 hours, the bitch should eat normally. If she refuses food for 24 hours, this is not serious, but any longer extension of 'fasting' is not normal, and veterinary advice should be sought. She should be offered food and drink in small amounts for the first two days. While she is feeding her puppies, the amount of food should be increased, often to three times the usual amount.

Should the bitch suffer because the nails of the puppies' front feet scratch her when they feed, these nails should be cut slightly shorter with sharp scissors.

In those breeds where the tail is docked or the dew-claws

Whelping

removed (qq.v.), this should be undertaken between the third and fifth day.

The bitch should be encouraged to take exercise.

The puppies should be handled each day to accustom them to human beings (*see* Section 2, 'Canine Behaviour Patterns').

Problems of the Post-Whelping Period (*see also* Eclampsia; Hand-Rearing of Puppies; Lactation, Defective; Lactation, Excessive; Mastitis)

INFECTION   Infection may occur when the resistance of the bitch is lowered following whelping. Probably the commonest cause is the retention of part of the afterbirth (q.v.) (the membranes enclosing the puppies before birth) within the bitch.

In many cases the bitch also suffers from mastitis (q v.).

The bitch has a raised temperature, will not feed her puppies and will not eat. Veterinary attention is essential. She should be kept warm and quiet, and the puppies removed temporarily (*see* hand-rearing of puppies). Any discharge should be wiped away from the vagina to prevent the bitch from licking and swallowing this. Give her water in small amounts at a time.

RETAINED AFTERBIRTH   This is a condition where part or all of the afterbirths are kept within the uterus. In most cases this causes little trouble, as the membranes degenerate and change into a brown liquid that runs away from the vulva. However, it is possible for infection to enter the body as a result (see above), or for part of the degenerating membranes to be reabsorbed and disturb the normal functions of the body.

If this condition is suspected, it is essential that veterinary advice be obtained.

For home treatment, if the bitch has a raised temperature, follow the instructions outlined in the section above headed 'Infection'. If the temperature is normal, she should be encouraged to move, and supplied with plenty of liquid. Naturally she should be kept warm. She should be examined for signs of mastitis (q.v.) and also for proof that she has an adequate milk supply for her puppies.

See also Lactation, Defective.

Weaning   This is partly a natural process, as puppies will start to eat the food put down for their dam at about 3 weeks of age. Milk can be lapped at about this time. Food should be gradually introduced from then on, at first to act as an additional source of

Whipworms

nourishment, then later to replace natural milk. By 8 weeks, the puppy should be capable of survival without the dam. If absolutely necessary, it is acceptable to remove a puppy at 6 weeks of age, but this may affect its development; such early removal should be avoided if possible.

See also Hand-Rearing of Puppies.

Unwanted Puppies   These should be taken away from the dam as soon as born. They should never be drowned, but should be humanely destroyed by a veterinary surgeon or one of the animal welfare societies.

Going to a New Owner   When a puppy is handed over to a new owner, some information about its upbringing should also be supplied. It is sensible to give a guide on the type of food being given, the times and amount for each meal, and suggestions for further feeding as the puppy grows. Where a record has been kept of the puppy's weight, this is useful for the new owner.

The new owner needs to have details and certificates of any inoculations or treatment the puppy has received.

For a pedigree puppy, the pedigree and registration certificate (if it has been registered) and signed transfer form, or the necessary papers (if it has not been registered) must be supplied.

Whipworms, *see* Parasites, Internal.
Worms, *see* Parasites, Internal.
Wounds, External   All external wounds can be divided into five types.

An *incised wound* is a clean cut by a sharp instrument, glass, etc.

A *lacerated wound*, where the skin and other parts are torn.

A *contused wound*, where the skin, etc. is torn and the edges are bruised. This often occurs when a dog is involved in a car accident.

A *puncture wound*, caused by a sharp point such as the claw of a cat, the bite of a dog, etc.

A *fistulous wound* is usually small, but penetrates deeply into the tissues. The exudate produced by an inflammatory reaction may drain away.

Treatment depends on the type of wound and also is influenced by other injuries if these exist. Antibiotics are required for all wounds, to prevent or control infection.

Incised wounds should be cleaned and then bandaged or sutured to draw the edges together. If haemorrhage is intense, a tourniquet (q.v.) should be applied until the dressing is in place. The wound should then be left undisturbed for 2 to 4 days and the dressings changed only when they become soiled, as the less the wound is disturbed, the quicker it heals.

A *lacerated wound* requires practically the same treatment. It must be thoroughly cleaned, and all shreds of loose or hanging pieces of skin removed. The wound is then dusted with a non-irritant, non-toxic, antiseptic powder, and bandaged. When healing has started and the wound appears dry, the bandage should be removed to allow air to the site. But care must be taken to ensure that the dog does not bite or scratch the site (*see* Licking).

In treating *puncture wounds*, the principal aim is to encourage healing from the bottom of the wound and not to allow the skin to heal before the lower part, otherwise an abscess may develop. The wound should be cleaned (with particular attention paid to the deeper parts). It should then be dried, dressed with acriflavine emulsion, and bandaged. This should be repeated two or three times a day.

Contused wounds are treated in the same way as a lacerated wound.

Fistulous wounds are often difficult to treat, and in many cases require removal of the basic cause.

GENERAL COMMENTS When bathing wounds, as a general principle, warm water with the addition of Epsom salts (a teaspoonful to 0·3 litres) is good for those where bleeding is slight; while the same solution, but cold, is better when there is considerable bleeding.

When a wound is the result of a bite, the risk of infection is great. Bathing should be prolonged and, where possible, the injury left unbandaged.

Always examine a wound to make sure that the cause of the injury is not still present; e.g. if a cut has been made by glass, it is possible that some of the glass still remains in the wound.

The hair around a wound should be clipped away so that the extent of the injury can be determined.

Puncture wounds are sometimes difficult to find. They can often be detected by stroking the skin, when the site is found to be slightly raised.

The possibility of the development of shock must be considered.

Dressings and bandages, once used, should not be re-used until

X-Rays

they have been washed and then boiled and dried. Any pad or dressing that has touched the wound itself should be thrown away.

X-Rays These are used to allow the examination of the internal structures of the body. The rays are passed through the body and to fall on an X-ray film. Parts of the ray are obstructed by the denser structures of the body and thus present a shadow on the plate when this is developed.

The denser the object outlined, the lighter it appears on the film.

The taking of such X-rays is a specialised procedure. In many cases it is necessary to give a dog a general anaesthetic beforehand.

The use of contrast liquids enables organs, etc. to be examined in this way although normally they would not be visible on an exposed film.

Two

The Dog in Health

The dog is not just a collection of muscle, nerves, bones and other structures. It is an animal that has likes and dislikes, that requires certain foods so balanced that they keep it healthy, that needs exercise to keep it fit and that has many inborn characteristics which should be understood. It is therefore sensible to include in a book which deals with the dog when unwell the needs of the healthy animal. When these are understood, the care of your dog, healthy or unfit, will become easier.

The requirements of the dog can be divided into three sections: those attributable to its nature and history—the so-called behaviour patterns; those needed when it is at home or in a kennel; and those dictated by food, its type and preparation and the effects of storage.

Canine Behaviour Patterns

It is now generally accepted that the wolf is the ancestor of the domesticated dog, this assumption being based on the similarity in the behaviour patterns of our dogs and the wolf. The wolf runs in packs, and in general each pack consists of a family group—the male, the female and their pups up to the age of about 2 years. The male asserts his authority to ensure that he leads the pack. He keeps the hierarchical position by aggression and is replaced only when a stronger, more intelligent male proves capable of taking over. Once the dominant male has asserted himself, aggression is no longer needed until a further challenge to his leadership occurs.

With the domesticated dog, Man has assumed the dominant position. Instinctively the male dog still possesses the desire to assert himself, and may attempt to dominate His human, especially during training. The owner's position is challenged and he must win. If the human dominance is only just maintained, the challenge

The Dog in Health

by the dog may be repeated. However, once human dominance is firmly asserted, the dog accepts this and the pack instinct ensures that he becomes part of human society with man as the 'pack leader'.

A puppy is born with all its instinctive behavioural patterns but with no knowledge of the external influences that will affect its life. It can neither see nor hear, but can taste, feel and smell. Its first knowledge of the world is the sensation of warmth from its dam, the taste of milk and the dam's smell. It quickly learns that these sensations do not exist elsewhere in its environment. It moves towards its dam and to the source of milk. It quickly learns that the licking by the bitch must be accepted. Left alone, this is the total of its experience until it can see and hear.

Even at this early stage, we can influence the puppy by handling. The warmth of the human hand, the smell associated with this, and the fact that the bitch does not object, are all noted and become part of the puppy's life.

Gradually it becomes aware of sounds. The eyes begin to open. Two new methods of obtaining information about the world have come into use. At first the puppy has to learn to use these new sense organs. As the days progress, it realises that sound comes from different directions and also learns to focus its eyes. By the time it is 17 or 18 days old, the puppy can receive ideas and is entering a period of maximum receptivity. It is about this time that it begins to move away from its dam, becomes inquisitive and starts to play.

The period between the third and the sixth week of age has an influence on the remainder of the dog's life. It is essential, during this period, for a puppy to have other puppies with which to play. Unless this companionship is available, the normal learning associated with play, including the development of normal body co-ordination and the ability to socialise with other dogs, is impaired. In the same way human handling, play and voice familiarisation are required to ensure a normal canine/human association.

Putting this another way, when a puppy is raised without canine companions it is not unusual for it to show aggression towards other dogs when it becomes older. In a similar way, a puppy raised without constant human association will often prove unacceptable if brought into a home as a house dog.

The Dog in Health

The puppy at 3 weeks of age is already beginning to take interest in food other than that supplied by its mother. By 6 weeks, this weaning process is advanced. It is at this stage that the puppy begins to feel that life is not entirely composed of enjoyable events. It starts to become more cautious and anxious in its attitude. Simple basic 'play training' becomes a possibility, as the puppy is anxious to please. This phase lasts for about 3 weeks, so that at approximately 9 weeks of age it undergoes a change in attitude, to become more actively cheerful again but less responsive to training.

From 3 months of age, the absorption of knowledge continues but it is not until mental development matures at about the sixth month that strict training can be expected to achieve good results.

Puppies must be allowed to see a variety of places and things as soon as they are inoculated. If they do not receive these impressions between 3 and 5 months of age, they often become nervous and excitable when later taken to unfamiliar surroundings—so much so that without this initial introduction at the receptive age to the stimuli of the outside world they may become completely unsuitable as household dogs and will be happy only when permanently kennelled.

In the wild, the wolf eats when it catches food. Its body is capable of digesting nearly everything it has hunted and it accepts that there will be days when no food is available. If this is used as a guide to the management of canine nutrition, it seems that an occasional 'fast' day, when food is withheld, would be acceptable and even advisable. However, one must not forget that the domesticated dog is anatomically different from its ancestors. We have only to look at the differences between various breeds to realise that any generalisation regarding feeding has not only to be amended to fit the requirements of each type of dog, but has also to be related to the previous feeding habits of each particular dog. Thus an adult Alsatian can be fed once a day and benefits from an occasional 'fast' day, but some of the toy breeds require a different feeding programme, with several meals a day and no fast period.

The comparison between the wolf and the present-day dog is endless. The mating of the wolf is carried out without any inhibitions. The mating of the dog can therefore be managed without any consideration of privacy or reduced light. On the other hand, whelping does include these conditions. Just as the wolf seeks

The Dog in Health

out a private lair where light is reduced when she is about to whelp, so the bitch should be supplied with suitable whelping quarters. Here, though, the owner has also to be considered and an additional light source must be available in case help has to be given.

It can be seen that a knowledge of the canine behaviour patterns helps the owner to understand his dog.

The Requirements of the Dog in the Home or Kennel

All dogs require a place where they can rest undisturbed. In the home, this may be under a table or in a corner. They need exercise, food, air, light and warmth. For the pet, this is usually no problem but for the kennelled dog, these factors have to be considered.

The following is a guide for the kennel owner.

Temperature within the kennel: for the dog, minimum 13°C and maximum 21°C (for humans, minimum 18°C); so the ideal general temperature should be 18–21°C.

Ventilation Healthy dogs require five air changes an hour, but this can be doubled without harm; the increased ventilation reduces the possibility of unpleasant odours within the buildings. Dogs should not be placed where there is a draught.

Noise should be controlled by dividing kennel blocks into small groups of kennels and by sound-proofing. Care must be taken to ensure that such divisions do not become dust and disease traps.

Kennel size A useful size is 2 × 1·25 metres. If dogs of only one breed or size are housed, the length of the dog can be used to determine the size of the kennel—1½ × 2 dog lengths should then be regarded as the minimum acceptable size.

Canine Nutrition

The ideal diet is a mixture that supplies all the elements needed for a dog's bodily development and functions. It should be completely balanced so that it provides all the nutrients and energy required by the body in the proper proportions. It must also be palatable enough to be eaten and in a form that is easy and pleasant to handle.

Where dogs are kept in kennels, the type of food used, its methods of preparation and the way it is stored have an important influence on the design of that part of a kennel devoted to food storage and preparation, so that it is sensible to decide what type of dietary management is to be used before the design of such a building is completed.

FOOD—ITS CONTENT, STORAGE AND THE EFFECT OF PREPARATION

All food contains water: thus root and green vegetables contain 75–90%; cereal grains—such as wheat—and biscuits about 10%. The amount of water contained can influence the keeping qualities. As a general rule, the heigher the percentage of water the poorer the stability of the food. Using cereal as an example, the normal percentage of water is about 10%; if this increases, the risk of deterioration also increases until at the level of 15–20% water mildew may develop.

Carbohydrates consist mainly of cellulose, starch and sugars. These differ in their digestibility. The starch has to be changed into sugars by enzymes in the digestive tract before it can be used. The sugars are readily absorbed, but the cellulose is quite indigestible. However, this cellulose, sometimes called *fibre*, is required in the food as it is needed to regulate the reabsorption of water in the lower part of the digestive tract.

The amount of carbohydrate needed is not fixed. It is an important source of calories because it is cheap and because it occurs in many food sources. It is generally considered that the maximum amount of carbohydrate in a complete food should be about 65%.

Cooked cereals can be utilised to an even greater extent, up to 80% of the diet, but this high level may cause diarrhoea in some dogs. Cooking reduces the indigestible part of the cereal. Although cereal can be stored for long periods, once it is cooked it can be preserved only by deep freezing or by being re-dried. Both processes require space and expensive equipment.

Protein is the nitrogenous part of the diet, composed of amino acids. There are about 23 of these but only 10 are indispensable, as if these are supplied to the dog it is able to make the remainder within his body.

Proteins that contain all the essential amino acids are called *complete*. Eggs, meat, milk, soya beans, peanuts and yeast contain these complete proteins. It is therefore possible to feed a dog adequately on a vegetarian diet if this is properly selected.

The Dog in Health

The amounts of the essential amino acids in the diet and their digestibility determine the true benefit of the protein eaten. Thus muscle and glandular organs are good, legume proteins reasonable, and other vegetable proteins vary in value.

The percentage of digestible protein is approximately: horse meat, 91; meat scraps, 86; fish meal, 88; liver meal, 88; blood meal, 78; soya bean meal, 86; linseed meal, 81. Limited heat does not reduce these values. Well cooked plant proteins have a higher digestibility than uncooked.

In practice, a minimum of 12% of the energy requirements of the adult dog should be supplied by protein, but many diets contain more than this to ensure that enough is available, as not all is usually digestible.

Most forms of meat and fish deteriorate rapidly with warmth, so that they soon become unfit to eat. If cooked they can be preserved for a short period, but the more practical method is to store meat or fish in the refrigerator, where it can be kept for days, or in the deep freeze, where it stays good for months. Space is the problem, as meat in bulk requires large, expensive cabinets.

Drying is a good method of preserving protein, but it takes longer to prepare when finally required. The dried product must be stored in a cool temperature, free from flies, dust and dirt, and away from moisture.

Fats are a major source of energy and are the most important means of energy storage within the body. The dog has a great capacity to absorb fat and can eat vast amounts of it, although this itself can cause problems.

The important points are: some fat is essential in the diet; this should be increased for an animal exposed to extreme cold; a deficiency will eventually lead to abnormal skin and hair development and an increase in the risk of skin infections; lard, bacon or vegetable fats, because of their high content of the type of fat that is essential for the dog, are better than other types.

Large amounts of fat in the diet reduce the amount of other food eaten and so stunt growth and may prevent the proper use of vitamin E within the body.

Fats and oils, if stored, should be kept cool and away from light and possible contamination. The action of light, etc., can cause rancidity, which in turn destroys the fat-soluble vitamins.

Minerals occur in most foods in sufficient quantities to keep dogs healthy. Calcium and phosphorus are needed in the proportions of 6 to 5, although this ratio can be widely varied without adverse effect if the dog gets adequate amounts of vitamins A and D in its diet.

When stored, minerals should be kept dry and clean.

Vitamins can be classed as water soluble or fat soluble.

The *water-soluble* vitamins are not easily stored within the body. Vitamin B deficiency often occurs with prolonged enteritis. Any dog that loses water because of this or due to vomiting requires additional vitamin B before it can utilise carbohydrate normally within its body.

The *fat-soluble* vitamins naturally require some fat in the diet to enable them to be absorbed. However, if additional oils, such as liquid paraffin, are given to a dog, these pass through the digestive tract and tend to absorb the fat-soluble vitamins and thus cause a deficiency.

Vitamins C and K are usually synthesised within the body and the normal healthy dog does not require them in the diet.

The preparation of a good diet takes common sense, time and care, but such 'home-made' foods are usually relatively inexpensive. 'Complete diets', either in tins or as dry pellets, are time-saving convenience foods.

Food is cooked (1) to sterilise, when contaminated products are used; (2) to increase palatability by improving the flavour and smell; (3) to break down the grain walls of starch and so increase the usefulness of carbohydrate; (4) to produce a gravy which can be used to increase the acceptability of other items of the diet. Prolonged cooking destroys vitamins. As a rough guide it is usual to cook (i.e. boil) for 15 minutes for each 500 grammes of food, taking this time from the point when the water boils.

Feeding a Dog

The amount of food required by any dog has to be determined by trial and error as each individual is different. Exercise affects the amount of food required—the more energy used while running about, the more food is required.

As a general rule, you should be able to feel your dog's ribs, but they should be covered by a thin layer of fat lying just under the skin. If a dog is overweight, it is usually because it is given too much energy-giving food. If this is reduced, or even eliminated, the body converts the fat into energy and so reduces weight.

The ideal is to weigh a dog regularly—perhaps monthly—and to feed approximately the same amount of food each day. If it gradually gains weight, then it is having too much to eat; if it is losing weight, it is not getting enough. But if it suddenly loses weight but is eating well, this might be due to some illness and veterinary advice is indicated.

As a rough guide, an adult dog requires about ½ oz (14 g) of food for every pound (454 g) it weighs. About two-thirds of this ration should be protein and the rest made up with cereal foods such as biscuits or meal. Table scraps can also be included—they give variety and a change of taste.

So, if we use this as a guide, a spaniel that weighs 30 lb (13·6 kg) would need 15 oz (426 g) of food daily, and this food should contain 10 oz (283 g) meat, 4 oz (112 g) cereal, and, possibly, 1 oz (28 g) table scraps. But as the cereal is an energy source, the amount supplied has to be adjusted to the individual. This diet might be deficient in vitamins and minerals and it is sensible to supply these as a palatable supplement in powder or tablet form.

Bones should be offered only if they are so large that the dog cannot break or splinter them. Uncooked large marrow bones are ideal, as they supply nourishment and help to strengthen the teeth. Dirty or old bones can be boiled (if they are to be used), but this must be done carefully, as they must be very well cooked (e.g. for 90 minutes). Small bones, whether cooked or not, and large bones, that can be chewed into pieces, are extremely harmful as they can cause obstructions in the digestive organs.

A bitch that is feeding her puppies requires extra attention to her diet. She must have more food, naturally (up to three times her normal diet), and this should be given as additional meals rather than by increasing the amount given at her normal feeding time. She should be given extra meat, vitamins and minerals—which really means increasing all types of food except carbohydrate.

The pregnant bitch requires twice her normal amount of food during the last half of pregnancy.

With any diet it is sensible to try to give variety, so that the

The Dog in Health

meal is made more interesting and the dog is learning to eat all types of food.

A number of 'complete diets' on the market supply all the nutritional requirements of the dog. These, not be to confused with ordinary tinned dog foods, are special diets which need no supplements and have been prepared under strict control. Some do specify the addition of carbohydrates, some do not, so the printed instructions should be carefully followed. They can be fed alone and will keep a dog healthy without trouble. It is important to remember that it is as bad to give too much as too little, and when these diets are used it is unwise to add any supplement unless so directed.

The normal adult dog should be fed once or twice a day. Always feed at the same time to encourage regular habits.

THREE IMPORTANT FEEDING RULES

1 Always use a clean food bowl.
2 Clean water must always be available.
3 Do not leave food down that is not eaten within a reasonable time.

FEEDING A PUPPY

The diet programme for puppies is more complex, as they are growing rapidly, and require frequent meals. The following programmes are suitable for puppies at different ages.

Aged 2–3 months—four meals a day.
Morning meal—minced meat or suitable tinned dog food plus granular dog meal, the latter given dry. The puppy will eat the meat first, then return at intervals to the rest.
Midday meal—milk with cereal, baby foods or breakfast cereals.
Late afternoon meal—as midday.
Evening meal—as morning meal, given an hour before bedtime to encourage the puppy to empty his bowels on his last trip outside.
Water must be available at all times.

The Dog in Health

Aged 3–6 months—three meals a day. Stop the late afternoon meal and gradually increase the quantity of meat and biscuits.

Aged 6–9 months—two meals a day, morning and evening.

From 9 months of age—one meal a day, unless you prefer to continue feeding twice daily.

See also Hand-Rearing of Puppies.

Three

Special Diets

In old age and in certain specific conditions, the types of food themselves may have to be altered. The following notes are intended as a guide, but it must be remembered that your veterinary surgeon may have to amend these depending on the condition of the dog.

The Old Dog

In old age the number of calories required is reduced, but the preparation of the food becomes more important. The amount of calcium and phosphorus may need to be increased because there is difficulty in maintaining the health of the bones of the body. Fat requirements are low; indeed excessive fat may interfere with the absorption of calcium. Protein is essential.

Carbohydrates should be cooked to break down the starch granules to help digestion, while vitamin supplements should be increased.

For the old dog you could prepare a diet of cooked cereals (oatmeal, wheat or rice) plus cooked meat, cottage cheese or boiled eggs, with added vitamins.

Having said all this, a vital proviso is that a dog that is aged but still eating its normal food should not suddenly be offered a new type of diet. It should be amended where needed.

Finally, old dogs require more frequent feeding; an additional meal a day without increasing the total daily amount helps digestion.

The Dog with a Weakened Digestion

Some dogs have a permanent weakness of their digestive system. Treatment is always indicated, but diet will also help. Bland but

Special Diets

appetising food, low in fibrous content, should be given. A plentiful supply of vitamin B is required. Fat should be supplied only in very small quantities.

Good foods include: meat, especially white meat, fish, cottage cheese, whole cooked eggs, cooked cereals. These should be given in small, frequent meals. In the same way, water should be offered 'little and often', but the total water intake should not be altered.

The Dog with Kidney Trouble

The diet should be nutritious and extremely palatable. Protein must be supplied, preferably white meat or fish. As a dog with severe kidney trouble often excretes a lot of protein in its urine, the amount it receives from its food must be increased.

Good foods include: white meat, rabbit, chicken, fish, cereal, milk, egg custard, cheese (in small quantities), hard-boiled eggs, vegetables, boiled rice and rice pudding.

Extra vitamin B should be supplied;—a yeast tablet two or three times a week is ideal.

The Diabetic Dog

This refers to the true 'sugar' diabetic condition caused by a shortage of insulin in the dog's body (*see* Diabetes Mellitus).

Exercise should be kept to the same amount each day to help treatment, and food should also be fed in the same daily quantities.

In the same way, the type of food should be constant. If a regular amount of food is given at regular times, the control of this illness may be more easily achieved.

'Diabetic' foods are ideal. Carbohydrate should be kept to a minimum. As treatment is usually a form of insulin given by injection, it is important to relate the feeding to the treatment given.

As a general principle, vitamin C should be supplied in large quantities—a number of reports of cases indicate that this condition can be controlled by the use of this vitamin.

For all the above conditions, one can buy diets prepared specifically for the illness concerned.

The Dog with a Bad Heart or Poor Circulation

Dogs with severe heart or circulatory conditions require, apart from veterinary treatment, food that has a low sodium content but a fairly high level of protein and carbohydrate. This is a rough guide, which may have to be varied on veterinary advice. Such dogs usually cannot excrete sodium and this encourages the fluid within the body to stay in the tissues, which, in turn, impedes the circulation. Therefore the diet should be low in salt, meat should be boiled and the water discarded, and 'titbits' should be avoided.

It is usually impossible to treat this condition by an alteration of the diet alone.

The Dog with a Wet Hindquarters Post-Urination

The thin, acrid boot of ammoniacy secretions can be spent from sebaceous tear cells, in ad that has a low moisture content at a fairly high level of protein and carbohydrate. This is a condition which is not must large in house cats, or occasionally adults which begin to cannot excrete sodium, and thus decrease the fluid volume of fit boot in tar by the tissue, which, in turn, suspends the concentration. Therefore, the diet should be above in salt water should be cooked and the water provided, and urinary absorbed be modified. It is usually inadvisable to treat this condition by appointment of the last given.

Four

The Dog when Unwell
Some Notes for the Dog-Owner

As a general principle for accident, illness or even old age, make sure that the dog does not become over-tired, and be especially careful in very hot or cold weather.

The sick dog needs constant attention, and wherever possible should have veterinary supervision. Dogs are like children—when they begin to feel better they try to do too much at once and this can cause a relapse. If a dog has lost its appetite and then starts eating again, it should not be given too much at once—little and often is better. Never let it drink too much at once. Don't encourage it to run about if it does not feel like doing this. In other words, build it up slowly.

But like all general principles, there can be exceptions, so follow veterinary advice, especially if the dog has had an operation.

Anaesthetics are a great boon and very safe, but care is needed as there is always a risk. You should never give a dog a drink when you are asked not to do so. During operations the owner has the hardest position of all those concerned, as he can only wait. Make sure you understand exactly what will be done, the advantages and problems, and what to expect afterwards.

Temperature

A dog's temperature is normally taken by inserting a short-nosed (stub-nosed) thermometer into the rectum. If the reading is higher than that expected (about 38·6°C, see below), shake the thermometer until the reading is low enough. Its surface should be coated with a thin layer of lubricant (olive oil, Vaseline or even butter). The instrument is then inserted so that about 4–5 cm (2 inches) are inside the dog. It should be left in place for 1 minute.

The normal temperature is approximately 38·6°C (101·5°F), but it can vary within 0·5° and still be within the normal range. It is

The Dog when Unwell

raised during infection, stress, or great exertion, and lowered in shock, some metabolic conditions, just before whelping, and when the dog is dying.

Giving Tablets

Sit the dog looking towards your right (if you are left-handed—looking towards your left). Place your left hand on top of its muzzle in front of the eyes and gently push the lips in onto the teeth. Using your right hand, open its mouth so that your left fingers push the lips between the teeth. It cannot then shut its mouth. Put the tablet at the back of its tongue, and gently push it further back using the right hand. Let the mouth shut, hold the head up but not too high, and rub the 'Adam's apple' until it swallows.

Remember to move firmly but gently—do not hurt the dog but make it feel that you have confidence in your ability to give tablets.

Of course, if it is eating, it may be easy to put the tablets into food as long as you are sure that it will eat it all up.

Giving Medicine

It is not necessary to open the dog's mouth. Hold its head slightly upwards and pour the liquid between the lips at the side of the mouth. The fluid runs down between the teeth and is swallowed. In some cases it is easier if one person holds the dog while another gives the medicine. The medicine should be given slowly to ensure that it is swallowed and does not cause choking.

Five

The First Aid Box

Every dog-owner should have a first aid box. This need not be an actual box, but can be a drawer, a shelf in a cupboard or a small medicine cabinet.

The number of things that could be kept for an emergency is inexhaustible. The following is a sensible list, but can be enlarged as you wish:

Cotton wool and bandages
Lint, gauze or clean white cloth
Washing soda crystals (can be given to cause vomiting)
A tape (*see* Muzzling a Dog)
Scissors
Elastoplast (a roll, not small pieces)
Liquid paraffin
Tweezers
Thermometer
Acriflavine emulsion or baby oil
A wound dressing powder
Potassium permanganate crystals
Epsom salts
Soluble aspirin
Bicarbonate of soda.

Six
Weights and Measures

This is an **approximate** guide to the metric and imperial system of weights and measures. For the use of measures in the home, it is more important to know the approximate than the precise equivalents of the two systems.

Fluids

1 fluid ounce = 30 ml
1 fluid drachm = 4 ml
15 minims   = 1 ml
1 litre   = 1·76 pints

Weight

1 kilogram = 2·2 lb
1 lb   = 453·6 grammes

Length

1 metre = 39·4 inches
1 yard = 0·91 metres

Household Measures

1 teaspoonful   =   5 ml   ⎫ These equivalents
1 dessertspoonful = 10 ml   ⎬ are *very* approximate
1 tablespoonful   = 15 ml   ⎪ and should not be
1 teacupful   = 140 ml   ⎭ used to measure drugs.

145

(01) 858.345 Ronnie